Heinz Schilcher

Phytotherapy
in Paediatrics

Phytotherapy in Paediatrics

Handbook for Physicians and Pharmacists

**With reference to Commission E Monographs
of the Federal Department of Health in Germany.
Includes 100 Commission E Monographs
and 15 ESCOP Monographs.**

By Prof. Dr. Heinz Schilcher, Berlin

Foreword by Prof. Dr. Dr. Hellbruegge

Revised and extended 2nd German edition
translated by A. R. Meuss, FIL, MTA

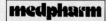

medpharm Scientific Publishers Stuttgart 1997

IMPORTANT NOTICE

All parties involved in the preparation and publication of this book have taken the greatest possible care to try to ensure that the information contained in it is correct and complete. However, no claims are made and no liability will be accepted in respect of such information. The medicines and dosages described in this book are offered as guidelines, subject in every case to current knowledge and research findings, to the manufacturer's current recommendations in the case of a proprietary product, and to the individual user's clinical judgement.

The use of general descriptive names, trade names, trademarks, etc. in a publication, even if not specifically identified, does not imply that these names are not protected by the relevant laws and regulations.

Title of original German edition:
Phytotherapie in der Kinderheilkunde. Handbuch für Ärzte und Apotheker
By Heinz Schilcher. 2nd edition.
© 1992 Wissenschaftliche Verlagsgesellschaft mbH
Birkenwaldstr. 44, D-70191 Stuttgart, Germany.
All rights reserved.

Translated from the 2nd German edition by A. R. Meuss, FIL, MTA

Die Deutsche Bibliothek – CIP - Einheitsaufnahme

Schilcher, Heinz
Phytotherapy in paediatrics : handbook for physicians and pharmacists ; with reference to Commission E monographs of the Federal Department of Health in Germany ; includes 100 Commission E monographs and 15 ESCOP monographs / by Heinz Schilcher. Foreword by Prof. Dr. Dr. Hellbruegge. Rev. and extended 2nd German ed. transl. by A. R. Meuss. – Stuttgart : Medpharm Scientific Publ., 1997
    Einheitssacht.: Phytotherapie in der Kinderheilkunde <engl.>
    ISBN 3-88763-026-2

Sole distribution rights for North America granted to:
Medicina Biologica, 2937 NE Flanders St., Portland, OR 97232, USA

The monographs bearing the mark (c) ESCOP are reprinted with kind permission of European Scientific Cooperative on Phytotherapy.

English language edition:
© 1997 medpharm GmbH Scientific Publishers,
Birkenwaldstr. 44, D-70191 Stuttgart, Germany
Printed in Germany

Foreword

One peculiar aspect of modern paediatrics is that phytotherapy for children has to be re-discovered. In my own childhood, treatment for children was entirely based on natural methods, from the much hated, itchy chest pack applied for all kinds of febrile conditions, various cough linctuses and antidiarrhoetics to chamomile and lime blossom tea. Mustard packs were still used when I was a clinical assistant at Munich University Children's Hospital, though only experienced nurses were permitted to apply them.

Antibiotics have caused this part of the paediatric armamentarium to fall into almost complete oblivion. In view of this, it is more than welcome to have Professor Schilcher, executive head of the Institute of Pharmaceutical Biology at Berlin's Independent University, present *Phytotherapy in Paediatrics* as a handbook for physicians and pharmacists.

This meets a need much felt among practising paediatricians – the desire to use natural methods in medicine: phytotherapy, homoeopathy, acupuncture and others.

Some academic experts in the field of paediatrics are dismissively critical of this development. It has to be remembered, however, that the need for "alternative" therapies has arisen in a generation of paediatricians who have had at least 5 years of strictly scientific training, followed by at least another 5 years of clinical training in hospitals where natural methods, including phytotherapy, are no longer used.

Schilcher's *Phytotherapy in Paediatrics* meets a real need among practising paediatricians and I am pleased to have been asked to write this Foreword.

Professor Theodor Hellbruegge
MD, hon. PhD, Munich

Preface

A look at current textbooks of phytotherapy and well-known books on natural medicine immediately makes it clear that paediatric practice is never given a separate chapter, despite the fact that phytotherapy seems ideally suited to this field. The same applies to scientific journals. Papers are occasionally published on the role of phytotherapy in geriatrics, but none on its potential usefulness and limitations in paediatrics. The Commission E Monographs include only four references to infants and children, although numerous drugs are suitable for paediatric use, some of which have been in continued use for a long time (e.g. fennel, sundew, thyme). Last but not least, several paediatricians stated in response to an enquiry that they only prescribe herbal medicines occasionally. It has to be added that on many occasions they believed phytotherapy to consist in the use of multi-ingredient homoeopathic medicines.

Herbal medicine, now also known as "phytomedicine", has tremendous potential in many areas, and these responses are therefore surprising, all the more so in view of the recently published *Medikamente und Kinder* (Medicines and Children) study commissioned by the Department of Health in North Rhine-Westphalia, Germany. The answers given by 2,000 mothers made it clear that children take medication even for minor indispositions, either of their own accord or at the instigation of parents. 28.6% of children aged 6 to 14 take a medicament at least once a month. When this representative study was presented by the Department, parents were advised to go back to the old "popular remedies", from compresses applied to the lower legs to the whole range of herbal teas. If we also remember that only 15% of childhood illnesses are treated by medical practitioners and 5% in hospital, it is easy to see the significance of proper self-medication, particularly in the case of children.

This book is designed to provide paediatricians, and also general practitioners, with recommendations and suggestions for the use of phytotherapeutic medicines. Phytomedicines can, of course, only be used in a limited number of conditions requiring treatment in infants, children and young people, but then with special justification. The book should thus be seen not so much as an alternative but as complementary to synthetic drug therapy [e.g. 70, 71]. A further aim is to provide pharmacists, frequently called on to give first-line information to parents, children and young people, with the knowledge required for responsible and medically justifiable self-medication. It has to be accepted that self-medication plays a major role in childhood illnesses.

The Commission E Monographs given in full in the Appendix provide "drugs legislation and scientific backing". Commission E has been appointed by the

Federal Department of Health in Germany to assess medicines based on plant substances for their indications, actions, side effects, etc. Individual Monographs may not expressly refer to use in paediatrics, but they provide additional information by giving the general indications, actions and posology.

The author is most grateful to the publishing house Wissenschaftliche Verlagsgesellschaft mbH, Stuttgart, for bringing his idea of publishing a book on paediatric herbal medicine to realization and for their constructive advice on the project. This book is a translation of the second German edition published in 1992. For the English edition it has been updated and revised where necessary. The ESCOP Monographs have been specially added to this English edition.

Special thanks are due to Professor Theodor Hellbruegge, Munich, for his Foreword, and to the paediatricians Dr Gabriele Heine, Berlin, and Dr Hugo Kroth, Munich, for their critical review of the original manuscript and their much appreciated support in finding the answers to specific medical questions.

Berlin, December 1996

Heinz Schilcher

Table of Contents

Chapter 1
Introduction and General Aspects

Chapter 2
Phytomedicines for External Use in Paediatrics

Chapter 3
Phytomedicines for Internal Use in Paediatrics

Chapter 4
References

Chapter 5
Commission E Monographs

Chapter 6
ESCOP Monographs

Abbreviations

DAC	German Medical Codex, 1979
Eur. P.	European Pharmacopoeia
GDR P.	Pharmacopoeia of former German Democratic Republic
Ger. P. 6	German Pharmacopoeia, sixth edition 1926
Ger. P. 10	German Pharmacopoeia, tenth edition 1991
Ger. P., Erg.-Bd. 6	Addendum to *Ger. P.* 6, *Addendum* reprinted 1953
Banz	Bundesanzeiger (German Federal Gazette)
iu	international unit(s)

Chapter 1

Introduction and General Aspects

1.1 Efficacy of Phytomedicines

In assessing the efficacy of a **herbal preparation**, physicians and pharmacists frequently face the dilemma that clinical results are not matched by scientific proof of efficacy based on clinical trials. The "conventional" school of medicine demands such proof and always seeks to provide it. This is to be expected in a discipline which has its epistemological origins in the rationalism and mechanistic views of René Descartes and the mathematical and physical laws of Isaac Newton, taken up by Paris and Berlin physiologists in the 19th century. In view of this historical fact it should not come as a surprise when opponents of "special therapies", to use a term from drugs legislation, consider natural medicines, which include herbal preparations, to be ineffective or placebos. Their views are presented in a paper by Schoenhoefer et al. in the journal *Paediatrische Praxis*. [69]

1.2 Phytotherapy and the Empirical Approach

A different view is taken in **empirical medicine**, a discipline with holistic orientation and enormous therapeutic potential. This includes all diagnostic and therapeutic methods which have not, or not yet, been scientifically examined and proven. Long-term observation and appropriate follow-up studies have confirmed their efficacy and made them both reproducible and teachable. E. Buchborn [20] writes: "Documented medical experience should rank equal with experiment, theory and observation." The high level of acceptance among patients and the growing therapeutic reputation of natural methods, including phytotherapy, among general practitioners – though unfortunately not many paediatricians – mean that empirical medicine must now be validated and active principles identified. The Federal German Government has set up a programme of "Research and Development to Serve Health" [21] which is intended to achieve this in stages. Commission E has drawn on documented reports from empirical medicine in producing its monographs (see pages 73–143), which is in accord with existing legal provisions and may also be seen to be scientifically acceptable.

1.3 The Role of the Physician and the Pharmacist as regards Scientific Phytotherapy in Paediatrics

The "scientific warfare" between protagonists of the "non-conventional" and "conventional" schools makes it important for **physicians** and **pharmacists** to distance themselves clearly from the lyrical indications given in popular and traditional medicine and obtain their information from the indications given in the Commission E Monographs and/or recent textbooks and handbooks of phytotherapy [22, 23, 90]. It is worth noting that a number of medical associations see phytotherapy as part of conventional rather than alternative medicine [24].

It is also important to know that uncritical acceptance of traditional reports and ancient herbals used as a revived materia medica [26] will do more harm than good to the cause of phytotherapy. Medical historian Prof. Keil of Wuerzburg warned against this at a scientific symposium held on the occasion of Prof. R. F. Weiss' 90th birthday. He went on to say that phytotherapy in particular was a field where medical and pharmaceutical historians found much to surprise them. Tracing traditions back to their source revealed not only errors in passing on information. More often than not a plant name used today referred to a completely different species in antiquity or the Middle Ages. According to Prof. Keil, exact botanical identification and description of the medicinal plant in question was the exception rather than the rule.

Scientific phytotherapy in paediatrics makes a number of specific demands on both **physicians** and **pharmacists**, especially if the preparation in question is also used for self-medication.

1 Taking account of the principle that pharmaceutical quality is a major factor in the efficacy of a herbal preparation, physicians should only prescribe preparations of high pharmaceutical quality, preferably standardized products, and pharmacists should take care to dispense this type of product. For this reason emphasis has quite deliberately been placed on standardized proprietary preparations in this book. The aim being to make this work useful in medical practice, attention is also drawn to commercially available drugs which may be of inferior quality.

2 Critical assessment of the **limits** of phytotherapy, especially with reference to indications recommended in certain lay publications [19] is another important aspect.

3 The wrong method of application, e.g. applying ointment containing menthol inside or immediately below the nostrils of infants, can cause immediate collapse (Kratschmer reflex). Pharmacists must therefore provide all relevant information. Knowledge of how to make a herbal infusion also tends to be lacking. Finally, the posology must be properly stated as it affects not only efficacy but also potential side effects.

1.4 Ground Rules for Childhood Phytotherapy, with Special Reference to Self-Medication

Before going into details of individual indications for phytotherapy, it will be necessary to consider some **basic** principles.

1 Before treatment is prescribed for infants and young children it is important to realize that the **rate of spontaneous recovery** from many acute conditions is much higher than it is in adults. Run-of-the-mill infections, for instance, most of them caused by viruses, will generally only persist a few days and do not require medical treatment. [27]

2 From the point of view of pharmacodynamics, most medicines have the same action in people of all ages, from the newborn to the aged. The required **dosage** and potential side effects tend to be very different, however. [27] Physicians and pharmacists should have a thorough knowledge of **age-related pharmacodynamics** and make use of this to a much greater extent than is generally done in practice. [27] The pharmacokinetics of many phytotherapeutic agents, especially those known to have gentle actions (*"mite"* medicines), tend to be unknown; particular attention must therefore be paid to pharmacodynamics and potential side effects.

3 A number of rules must be observed with self-medication, especially in paediatrics.

- Try to establish the cause before using self-medication.
- Do not take any medicine at random but look for one that is specific.
- Do not take several medicines at the same time.
- Use the lowest possible dose to deal with symptoms. "The more you take the better the effect" is not the right idea!
- As far as possible, relate treatment to the rhythms of the disease process (chronopharmacology).
- Only use self-medication in the short term. If you treat yourself for any length of time real problems may go unrecognized.
- If there is no improvement after taking the medicine for several days to treat what may be familiar symptoms, go and see a doctor.
- Clouding of consciousness, disorientation or other disorders of consciousness, paraesthesia, paralysis, cardiac arrhythmias occurring for the first time, indefinite pain in the chest or abdomen and indefinite symptoms which go beyond the limit of "everyday" problems require proper medical attention.

4 In paediatrics, phytotherapy is of **value** primarily because many phytomedicines have a relatively good **benefit-risk** ratio. The actions of many combinations of natural compounds (e.g. essential oils, bitter principles, flavonoids, tannins, saponins, mucilages) and of many individual such compounds (e.g. chamazulene, camphor, bisabolol, menthol, rutin) have been experimentally established and/or clinically confirmed, with side effects minimal if not negligible. The Commission E Monographs (see Ap-

pendix) provide "official" confirmation of both the efficacy and the low level of side effects of all medicinal agents recommended in this book.

Secondly, many if not all of these agents are of value in paediatrics because of their **gentle ("mite") action**. [1] It is very often the case that gentle, or weak medicinal actions are perfectly adequate in the treatment of childhood diseases.

Thirdly, the **methods of administration** (e.g. inhalation, baths, ointments, syrups) commonly used in phytotherapy are particularly acceptable to children.

This, and the cooperation of mothers or carers who are generally much in favour of phytotherapy, provides for **good compliance**.

The fifth argument in favour of phytomedicines in paediatrics is that fact that a number of these may be used for **causal**, and not merely symptomatic, treatment.

Finally it is worth pointing out that phytomedicines are as a rule **less expensive** than comparable synthetic drugs, especially if medicinal teas, tinctures, inhalations, ointments, etc. are prescribed.

1.5 Formulation of Medicinal Teas (Species)

Mixtures of medicinal agents (species) are more commonly prescribed in phytomedicine than single drugs. There are a number of reasons for this. [77, 78] A medicinal tea is made up as follows:

1 The **remedium cardinale**, the basic medicinal agent – for a laxative tea, for instance, one or more anthranoid drugs (senna leaves, frangula bark, etc.).

2 The **adjuvans**, drugs to enhance or complement the action of the basic medicinal agent or reduce undesirable side effects. Thus drugs with carminative (anise, caraway or fennel seed) and/or spasmolytic properties (chamomile flowers, silverweed) may considerably reduce the undesirable side effects like gripes of anthranoid drugs.

3 The **constituens, corrigens** and **colorants**. To prevent the tea separating into its components, up to 20% of plant material with no or limited medicinal action which, however, must be very hairy is added to the mixture. Raspberry leaves are frequently used as a "filler", for example. To ensure compliance, a medicinal tea should, or indeed must, be reasonably palatable. This is particularly important in paediatrics. Widely used "aromatics" are bitter orange peel, orange blossom, hibiscus flowers, peppermint leaves, etc. Finally a tea must also inspire confidence and look interesting. Colorants like cat's foot, cornflower, mallow, marigold flowers, etc., are used for that purpose.

A medicinal tea thus contains at least 4, but generally 5−10 components.

Prescribing Medicinal Teas

The prescription (written direction for preparation and administration) of species is based on the following method:

I *Nomen aegroti* (patient's name):

_____

II *Superscription:* The symbol R_x or the word Recipe, meaning "take"

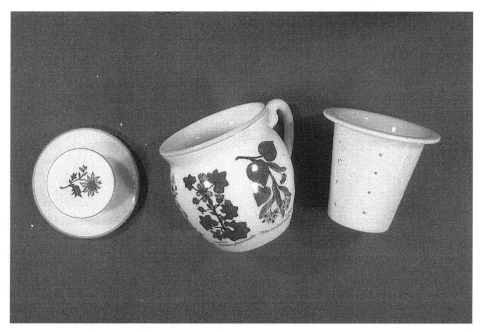

Fig. 1. Special cup with strainer for medicinal teas

III *Inscription:* Details and quantities of ingredients
Birch leaves, minced, or
Betulae folium conc. = concisus
20.0 g
Golden rod herb, minced, or
Solidaginis herba conc. 20.0 g
Java tea leaves, minced, or
Orthosiphonis folium conc. 20.0 g
Bearberry leaves, minced, or
Uvae ursi folium conc. 30.0 g
Peppermint leaves, minced, or
Menthae piperitae folium conc.
10.0 g
IV *Subscription:* Directions for compounding
Misce fiat species urologicae (abbr.: M. f. spec.) or M. D. S. = misce, da, signa (mix, give, mark)
V *Signa:* Mark
Bladder and kidney tea
1 tablespoon to 1 cup of water, as an infusion, 3 x daily after meals, to be taken at about body temperature.
VI *Nomen medici:* Doctor's signature

1.6 Method of Producing Medicinal Teas

1.6.1 Infusion
(Latin *infusum*, abbr. inf.)

Infusions are not normally produced according to the directions given in the *German Pharmacopoeia (Ger. P.)* 8. *Ger. P.* 10 no longer contains such directions.

The correct method is to transfer the required amount of the minced, or cut-up, drug to a suitable container, add 150−200 ml of boiling water, cover the container and leave to infuse for about 10 minutes, after which the tea is poured through a tea-strainer whilst still hot. Special herbal-tea cups of the type shown in Fig. 1 help to simplify the procedure.

Fruits containing volatile oils, e.g. fennel, anise, caraway, dill, parsley and juniper fruits, need to be crushed or bruised (Latin: *contusus*) before the hot water is added.

Infusions made with drugs which do not contain volatile oils, e.g. hawthorn flowers and leaves, may be simmered on a low flame for an additional 5 minutes or so. This applies particularly to flavonoid drugs. Infusions of bitter herbs on the other hand must not be boiled as prolonged heating reduces the bitter index.

1.6.2 Decoction
(Latin *decoctum*, abbr. decoct.)

Again, consumers should not follow the directions given in the *Ger. P.* 8. De-coctions are normally made of woody, bark and root parts of plants. The method is to put the prescribed amount (tsp or tbs) in a suitable container, add about 200 ml of hot water, keep hot (above 90 °C) on a small flame for 30 minutes and pour the hot decoction through a tea-strainer.

1.6.3 Maceration
(Latin *maceratio*, abbr. mac.)

In just a few cases (bearberry leaves, marshmallow root, mistletoe herb, senna leaves) extracts are made at room temperature for galenical reasons (e.g. high starch content of marshmallow roots) or to improve tolerance (e.g. of bearberry leaves). The method is to place the minced material in cold water, cold boiled water if required, and leave to stand for 8 hours, stirring occasionally, before straining. The resulting extract should be brought briefly to the boil before it is taken, to kill any microbes present.

Chapter 2

Phytomedicines for External Use in Paediatrics

2.1 Caring for the Sensitive Skin of Infants and Young Children

Care of sensitive skin is particularly important in

- infants,
- children who are immobilized or confined to bed,
- handicapped children with cerebral palsy,
- chronically sick or seriously ill children with faecal and urinary incontinence.

The plant-based preparation of first choice is a suitable preparation of **chamomile flowers, Matricariae flos (*Eur. P.*)** from *Chamomilla recutita* L. Rauschert. "Suitable" preparations are extracts from chamomile flowers with sufficiently high concentrations of **antiinflammatory principles** (e.g. Tinctura Chamomillae). Such principles are said to include

- (−) α-bisabolol
- chamazulene or matricine
- apigenin > luteolin > quercetin. Apigenin is the more effective flavonoid.

An ethanolic extract containing adequate amounts of lipophilic (volatile oil) and hydrophilic (flavonoids) principles is more suitable than a purely aqueous extract, even if this has been produced from chamomile flowers *Eur. P.*

The best possible preparation to use for sitz-baths and for local applications is an aqueous infusion of chamomile flowers *Eur. P.* (2 tablespoons for a full baby's bath or sitz-bath), reinforced with 10−20 ml of a proprietary standardized ethanolic chamomile preparation (see p. 21). The use of extracts made from "chamomile for baths" (see Fig. 2) is not recommended, as the concentration of antiinflammatory principles is minimal. It is also known that strict hygiene regulations are not always observed in the gathering and preparation of these inferior products.

Chamomile ointments, either proprietary (see p. 21), individually dispensed or made up according to prescription (see p. 20 and 21) and/or chamomile oils obtained from pharmacists are excellent for **dry** and sensitive **baby skin**.

Suggested Formula for Oleum Chamomillae

1 Volatile oil of chamomile flowers 8.0 g
   Neutral fatty oil   ad 100.0 g

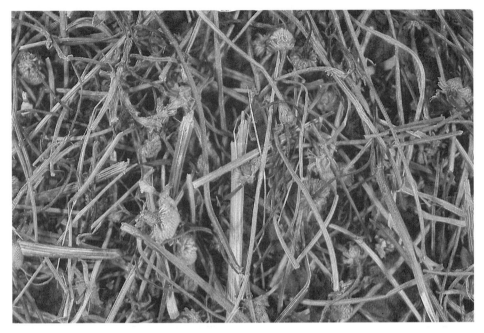

Fig. 2. Chamomile quality for baths

2 Standardized ethanolic tincture of chamomile (ethanol content 40 % v/v) (e. g. Kamillosan®) 5.0 g
Neutral fatty oil
(e.g. Miglyol®) ad 100.0 g
(Note: Volatile oil of chamomile is commercially available at approx. DM 2,000.00/kg).

The action of witch hazel leaves and bark (Hamamelidis folium and Hamamelidis cortex from *Hamamelis virginiana* L.) is due to another class of active principles, the tannins. The astringent effect of witch hazel gallic acid and catechin tannins creates a form of "protective layer" on the sensitive skin of infants and young children. Gallic acid tannins, in particular, which are hydrolysable, also have additional antiinflammatory activity. The volatile oil present in addition to the tannins in witch hazel leaves and branches has similar activity (see Commission E monograph).

Hamamelis baths
For 1 full bath make a decoction (in approx. 250 ml of water, about 10 minutes on a low flame), using about 10 g of witch hazel leaves or bark. Good results have also been obtained with Hamamelis Water BPC (3 tablespoons to a sitz-bath).

For dry skin, hamamelis ointments may be used (see p. 21), either proprietary brands or your own prescription: e.g. R_x Extractum Hamamelidis fluidum
5.0 g
Unguentum molle ad 30.0 g
or (Unguentum emulsificans
aquosum ad 30.0 g)
Calendulae flos preparations are best in form of proprietary products.

Aloe preparations (from *Aloe vera*), which are now widely used in cosmetics, are less suitable for children because of the bitter taste. Even with topical use it is not possible to prevent mouth contact.

2.1.1 Proprietary Products

APS Hautbad med.,
Kamillosan® liquid, Kamille® (Spitzner) solution, Perkamillon® liquid.
Chamo® ointment (Buerger, Ysat), Kamillosan® ointment, Hamasana® ointment, Hametum® ointment, Perkamillon® ointment, Calendula ointment Helixor
Freiöl®, Caelo-Kamillenöl (= Chamomillae aetheroleum *Ger. P.* 10).

2.2 Inflammatory skin conditions

Phytotherapy is primarily indicated for the following:

- nappy rash (dermatitis glutealis infantum syn. dermatitis ammoniacalis),
- milk crust (dermatitis seborrhoica),
- neurodermatitis (dermatitis atopica),
- exfoliative dermatitis,
- inflammatory changes in the genital area, e.g. vulvitis.

It is of course self-evident that phytotherapy can merely be supportive therapy on these indications, but an extremely useful one, essentially offering symptomatic improvement.

2.2.1 Nappy Rash

The question as to whether a dermatitis glutealis infantum can be effectively treated with phytomedicines only, at the same time changing the method of using nappies, will depend on the severity and type of microbial infection (yeasts and/ or staphylococci, among others) and the degree of inflammation. Supportive treatment using the chamomile flower preparations given below will always serve a purpose, however.

Sitz-bath. Dissolve 1 tablespoon Extractum Chamomillae fluidum or of a standardized proprietary chamomile preparation in 1-2 litres of warm water, preferably water that has been previously boiled.

Local application. Dilute the abovementioned ethanolic chamomile extracts 1 : 4 with water before gently dabbing to the inflamed areas.

Chamomile ointment. Apart from using proprietary products, "Unguentum Chamomillae" may be formulated as follows:

Extr. Chamomillae fluidum or proprietary ethanolic extract
e.g. Kamillosan® or Kamille Spitzner
8.0 g
Ungt. Zinci or Zinci pasta mollis
ad 50.0 g

Chamomile and sulphur ointment
Sulphur praecipitatum 3.0 g
Extr. Chamomillae fluidum or
Kamillosan® solution 10.0 g
Oleum Jecoris 20.0 g
Zincum oxidatum 30.0 g
Adeps lanae ad 100.0 g

Chamomile baby powder
Extr. Chamomillae fluidum or proprietary ethanolic extract 5.0–10.0 g
Talc or zinc oxide ad 100.0 g

Another used medicinal plant in this area is **wild pansy** (*Viola tricolor*, L.) Aqueous extracts of the herbaceous parts (Violae tricoloris herba) have emollient properties. They are used in sitz-baths, for lavage and in compresses. A tea (1 tablespoon to 1 cup of water = ca 200 ml) is particularly useful for softening milk crusts. For a sitz-bath, pour 1 litre of boiling water over 2–3 tablespoons of the herb and leave to infuse for about 15 minutes. Strain and add to the bath water.

2.2.2 Milk Crust, Neurodermatitis

Phytotherapy may also be used to relieve the troublesome, often tormenting symptoms of seborrhoeic dermatitis (milk crust) in the first months of life, and atopic dermatitis (chronic eczema = neurodermatitis) from about the 5th month. Treatment of these essentially constitutional conditions requires parents not only to feel affection for these "small patients" and show patience and perseverance, but above all to know how **local skin lesions** and the troublesome irritation are best treated.

Local treatment will need to be handled individually, depending on the type of skin defect. Dry areas may be kept supple with **"chamomile oil"** or a **chamomile cream**. Inflamed areas, papules or itching, weeping, scaling crusts mainly on the cheeks and hairy scalp ("cradle cap, milk crust") are treated by dabbing on dilute tincture of chamomile flowers (1:4). In severe cases a short course of glucocorticoid therapy may be unavoidable. Weeping areas are dried out with a **chamomile zinc ointment**.

In a recent double blind trial [91] the efficacy of a standardized **hamamelis ointment** (see p. 23) was compared with that of an ointment containing bufexamac in the treatment of neurodermatitis. Overall there were no signifi-cant differences, with marked improvement in the symptoms from both ointments.

Pruritus or **skin irritation** is relieved by **oat straw baths** made with 50–100 g of **Avenae stramentum** (see Commission E monograph) to a full bath, or by a **bran bath**. The irritation is also relieved by washing with "peppermint or mint oil water", i.e. 5–10 drops of peppermint or mint oil "dispersed" in 1 litre of water by vigorous shaking. Small amounts of the volatile oil, above all up to 28% of cooling menthol, dissolve in the water. [28] Warning: Do not use pure mint oil or tincture.

A final phytotherapeutic measure would be to give **evening primrose** oil by mo uth. A number of placebo-controlled and cross-over trials have shown this to give subjective and objective improvement. The results are not dramatic, however. Taking evening primrose oil evidently corrects the delta-6-desaturase deficiency, clearly one step in complex therapy. Borage seed oil has the highest concentration of gamma linolenic acid.

2.2.3 Exfoliative Dermatitis

Oat straw baths are recommended in phytotherapy, again mainly to reduce the irritation. The use is established in the Commission E Monograph. Boil 50–100 g of Avenae stramentum for about 30 minutes in 2 litres of water, strain and add the liquid to the bath water.

2.2.4 Inflammation in the Genital Region

Vulvitis may be treated with chamomile sitz-baths using 10–20 ml of chamomile tincture to about 5 litres of water. Sitz-baths using tinctures of Millefollii herba (yarrow) or even better yarrow flowers (Millefolii flos, from *Achillea millefolium* L.) are also suitable. For adequate antibacterial and antiinflammatory activity, use not less than 10 ml tincture of the herb, or even better the flowers, per sitzbath. It is important for the tinctures to have a high azulene content.

2.2.5 Proprietary Products

APS® Hautbad med, Kamillosan® liquid, Kamille® (Spitzner) liquid, Perkamillon® liquid, Salus® Schafgarbentropfen (yarrow drops)
Hametum® ointment, Schupp® Peppermint oil
JHP-Rödler Japanisches Heilpflanzenöl (mint oil), Röwa Minz K Heilpflanzenöl (mint K herbal oil), Epogam® Evening Primrose Oil, Glandol®

Phamacopoeia Monographs

Peppermint oil (Menthae piperitae aetheroleum *Ger. P.* 10), Mint oil (Menthae arvensis aetheroleum *Ger. P.* 10), Chamomile flower oil (Oleum chamomillae *Ger. P.* 10).

2.3 Wounds, Burns

2.3.1 Treatment of Wounds

Grazes are particularly common in children. Instead of the usual primary application of iodine tincture or an antiseptic such as Merfen Orange (phenylmercuric acetate), both of which may cause allergic reactions, ethanolic tinctures of **chamomile** or **yarrow flowers** are highly

suitable for paediatric use, especially if used as fluidextracts or standardized proprietary products (see p. 23). Both phytomedicines have been shown to have bacteriostatic and antiinflammatory actions (see also Commission E Monographs). For infants and young children, dilute 1:1 or 1:2, so that they won't "sting".

There is both experimental and clinical proof of efficacy for **mint oil** in the treatment of grazes.[32] It may be used undiluted for adults, though only a few drops for external application, and a 1 + 9 dilution is recommended for children. A suitable diluent is a neutral fatty oil such as Miglyol®.

Arnica tincture should not be used with children, unless made from **Spanish** arnica flowers.[31] It has been known for some years that the sesquiterpene lactone esters of the **helenalin** type (Fig. 4) may cause **contact dermatitis**.

The **dihydrohelenalin compounds** that are the main constitutions of arnica flowers of Spanish provenance* have much lower or no allergenic potential. This is due to absence of the exocyclic methylene group, a group with nucle-

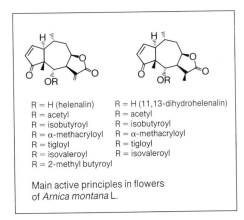

R = H (helenalin)   R = H (11,13-dihydrohelenalin)
R = acetyl   R = acetyl
R = isobutyroyl   R = isobutyroyl
R = α-methacryloyl   R = α-methacryloyl
R = tigloyl   R = tigloyl
R = isovaleroyl   R = isovaleroyl
R = 2-methyl butyroyl

Main active principles in flowers
of *Arnica montana* L.

Fig. 3. Sequiterpene lactones in Arnicae flos

---

* Used in Kneipp® Arnica Ointment.

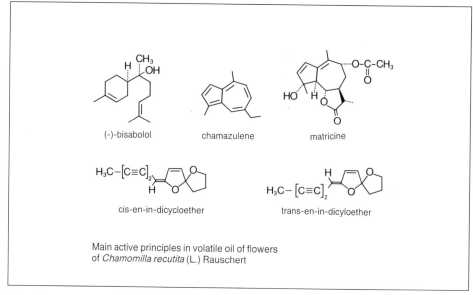

Main active principles in volatile oil of flowers of *Chamomilla recutita* (L.) Rauschert

Fig. 4. Constituents of the volatile oil in Matricariae flos

ophilic properties that are liable to react with amino groups and SH groups of skin proteins.

The arnica flowers normally seen on the market have the highest allergenic potential of the daisy family (Asteraceae), according to Hausen, B. M.[29] It is best for children not to come in contact with the arnica contact allergens, despite the fact that arnica tincture is a popular family medicine for treating injuries.

According to Hausen, [33] preparations of "true" chamomile can be used without risk of contact dermatitis, despite occasional reports to the contrary. Hausen et al. [34] have been able to identify the contact allergen in poor-quality chamomile preparations that may cause contact dermatitis. It is the linear sesquiterpene lactone **anthecotulide** (Fig. 5), large amounts of which are found in corn chamomiles, especially stinking chamomile (*Anthemis cotula* L.). The new Degumille® and Manzana® types of chamomile* and several European chamomiles were found to be free from anthecotulide. Mere traces were found in trade samples from Chile and Argentina, [33] according to Hausen et al. [34] not enough for contact sensitization. Hausen also points out that an epicutaneous test positive for chamomile does not necessarily indicate allergy to chamomile. The positive result may be due to a cross reaction in someone allergic to chrysanthemum.[33] Our own investigations on cross allergies among members of the daisy family (Asteraceae) are still at the experimental stage.

Wounds may also be treated with a range of plant-based ointments, creams or gels.

---

* Degumille® is a diploid (= 2 n), Manzana® a tetraploid (= 4 n) chamomilla cultivar.

Calendula ointment, produced from **Calendulae flos** (from *Calendula officinalis* L.) merits first place in the list. The Commission E Monograph lists under Indications: "Wounds, including those with poor healing tendency". Calendula ointments of high pharmaceutical quality are made with ethanolic and/or oily extracts of ligulate florets only.

Other useful preparations are **chamomile ointments, echinacea ointments** and galenical preparations containing **Peru balsam** (for proprietaries, see p. 26). Peru balsam should not be used if there is a marked allergic disposition. The same applies to ointments containing **propolis**, which have been widely used in recent times. The indications given for **Peru balsam** in the Commission E Monograph are: "External application for infected wounds with poor healing tendencies, burns, bedsores, chilblains, leg ulcers, pressure sores from prostheses, and haemorrhoids". "Allergic skin reactions" are listed as side effects. For paediatrics, the reference to the **antiparasitic** action of Peru balsam is of interest. This was primarily demonstrated for itch mites.

Wound ointment to support treatment of wounds with poor healing tendency:

R_x Equiseti decoct.
aquosum 10%   80.0 g
Eucerin anhydricum   ad 200.0 g
M. f. ungt. D. S. Apply thinly once a day.

Wound ointment
R_x Chamomile oil
(Chamomillae aetheroleum)   1.0 g
Panthenol   2.0 g
Vitamin A palmitate   200,000 g
Echinacea mother tincture   2.0 g

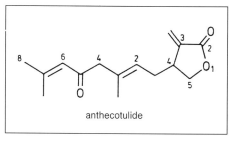

Fig. 5. Anthecotulide, the allergen in *Anthemis cotula*

Ungt. emulsificans
aquosum   ad 50.0 g

2.3.2 Burns

Hypericum oil is the first choice for treating burns. It is an oily extract of Hyperici herba (botanical name *Hypericum perforatum* L.). Indications: "1st degree burns" also in the Commission E monograph. The pharmaceutically valuable "red oils" are produced from stripped-off leaves and flowers only, which means high hypericin and pseudohypericin concentrations. The thin-layer chromatogram shows marked differences between different commercial products (Fig. 6).

Before hypericum oil is applied, the scalded or burned areas should be cooled immediately at the accident site by immersing in cold water or pouring this over for several minutes. Local treatment with Oleum Hyperici may then follow. Place sterile gauze soaked in the "red oil" on the burned areas. Renew the oil dressing after about 10 hours. This phytotherapeutic measure will not only cause the wound to heal rapidly but also prevent unsightly scars from developing.

Hypericum oil is also suitable for treating sunburn. Avoid direct sunlight for some hours after application (see Monograph in Appendix).

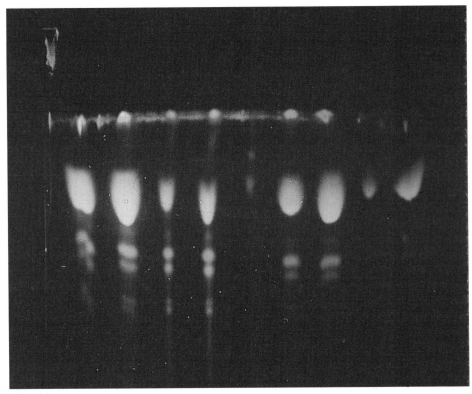

Fig. 6. Thin-layer chromatogram of Hypericum extracts with different hypericin contents

2.3.3 Proprietary Preparations

Kamillosan® liquid, Kamille® (Spitzner) liquid, Perkamillon® liquid, Kneipp® Arnica ointment, Echinacin® ointment; Echinacea ointment Fides, Hewekzem novo ointment, Peru-Lenicet® ointment, Jukunda® Rotöl, Kneipp® Johanniskraut-Öl N. (St John's wort oil)

Monographs

Chamomile flowers fluidextract (Extractum Chamomillae fluidum, *Ger. P.*, Erg.-Bd. 6), Chamomile flower tincture (Chamomilla tinctura, *Austr. P.*, Erg.-Bd. 6), yarrow flower tincture (Millefolii tinctura, *Ger. P.*, Erg.-Bd. 6)

2.4 Contusions, Crush Injuries, Sprains, Dislocation, Strain Injuries

Comfrey pastes and **ointments** have proved highly effective in the treatment of blunt traumas, as is well known from the fields of sports and industrial medicine. The pharmaceutical preparations are made from **comfrey root, Symphyti radix** (botanical name *Symphytum officinale* L.). Active principles are thought to be allantoin (the crude drug contains up to 2%) and mucilage (up to 30%). The root also contains traces of pyrrolizidine alkaloids (PAs) but these are not involved in the medicinal action. Allantoin accelerates cell regeneration and has antiinflammatory properties. The mucilage has local emollient actions and binds water, which makes it suitable for use in heat-holding compresses. The good to excellent results the author has seen in himself and many people he has treated are clearly due to other active principles as well. The German Commission E Monograph provides the following indications: "Contusions, crush injuries, sprains, dislocation, strain injuries". PAs may be a risk factor, but having carefully studied the literature on pyrrolidizine alkaloids and for several years the scientific information on Symphytum, also taking account of the expert opinion of Dr Lucthy, Zurich, we are of the opinion that for topical applications of Symphytum preparations the benefits outweigh the risk. This applies particularly to preparations made from Symphytum "types" with low pyrrolizidine alkaloid levels. Analysis of large numbers of individual plants has shown the alkaloid content of fresh plant material to be between 14 and 2,200 mg/kg. A special safety measure that could be introduced for paediatric use would be to demand determination of pyrrolizidine alkaloid levels or of limiting values (e.g. 50 μg of alkaloids/100 g of product is feasible and acceptable). Limitation to a daily dose of 100 μg of pyrrolizidine alkaloids with 1,2-unsaturated necine structure including their N oxides should provide adequate safety even for paediatric use. In conclusion, let it be emphasized once more that there is no phytotherapeutic drug that can replace Symphytum preparations for topical use, especially as a paste for rapid-action compresses (for proprietary preparations, see under 2.4.1).

Blunt traumas and especially painful **haematomas** may also be treated to good effect with **horse chestnut ointments** or **gels**. The plant extracts used for these are usually inspissated aqueous extracts of **Hippocastani semen** (botanical name *Aesculus hippocastanum* L.) with aescin levels showing considerable variation (α-aescin, β-aescin, cryptoaescin, aescinols). The type of ointment base used is important for efficacy, as is the use of occlusive dressings. The Commission E monograph suggests the following indications for horse chestnut seed preparations: "Posttraumatic and postoperative soft tissue swelling." Only standardized proprietary products should be used (see under 2.4.1).

Pain is relieved by massaging in a few drops of **peppermint** or **mint oil** or the use of menthol sprays, though these should **not** be used on infants. Gas chromatography shows only very minor differences between the different products based on *Mentha arvensis* L. var. *piperascens* Holmes ex Christy.

Prescriptions may be made out for

peppermint oil (Menthae piperitae aetheroleum, formerly Oleum menthae piperitae) or mint oil (Menthae arvensis aetheroleum). Use only 4−6 drops for external application.

2.4.1 Proprietary Preparations

Kytta-Salbe®, Venostasin® ointment, Venotrulan® ointment, Reparil® gel
JHP Rödler Heilpflanzenöl and others.

Monographs

Peppermint oil *Ger. P.* 10 (Menthae piperitae aetheroleum), mint oil *Ger. P.* 10 (Menthae arvensis aetheroleum).

2.5 Herpes

Infection with herpes simplex virus type I and II is very common even in early infancy. Following contact with a carrier, the virus generally penetrates the mucocutaneous barrier through the tiniest of mucosal lesions. The border between lips and oral mucosa is the preferred site for herpes simplex virus type I (herpes labialis) infection, the genital region for herpes simplex type II (herpes genitalis).

Phytotherapy initially concentrates on symptomatic treatment (local redness, vesicles, swelling, etc.). Suitable preparations are anti-inflammatory ointments and tinctures of chamomile flowers, calendula flowers and yarrow flowers. A standardized **extract of balm leaves** in

Lomaherpan® ointment is said to have additional virostatic properties. [83]

"Lip care" is provided by an Echinacin® lipstick.

2.6 Eye Conditions

Conjunctivitis is one of the most common conditions diagnosed in paediatric opthalmology.[70] The incidence is particularly high in cities and industrial areas. The main symptoms, which also respond to phytotherapy, are foreign body sensation, burning, sensation of pressure around the eye, irritation, heavy lids and fatiguability.[70]

Herbal preparations can however only be used to treat conjunctivitis due to chemical or physical causes (conjunctivitis simplex) and the condition known as "spring catarrh", which affects about 70% of boys and young males in Europe.

Extracts of **eyebright** (Euphrasiae herba) and **Aqua Foeniculi** are recommended for washes and eye baths. To make an eyebright extract, infuse about 2 g of the dried plant drug for 10 minutes in 150 ml of water and filter hot, preferably using a sterile membrane filter. Eyebright eye lotion, formerly made according to the above directions, should be produced in a pharmacy today, using water for injections and sodium chloride plus the legally required preservative. Eye lotions should be approximately isotonic with lachrymal fluid, which is achieved by adding sodium chloride. The **negative** Monograph passed by Commission E is essentially designed to deal with hygiene problems that arise when lay people make up eye lotions for self-medication. The filtered extract is applied several times daily, using an eye bath.

Fennel water, obtainable as Aqua Foeniculi from pharmacists, is used in a similar way.

A small number of proprietary products have proved useful in treating conjunctivitis simplex in children and young people. They are Berberil® drops, Salus Augenbad (eye lotion) and "Iso-Werk" Augentropfen (eye drops). Berberil® is not a purely phytotherapeutic drug. "Iso-Werk" Augentropfen combine Aqua Foeniculi, the main constituent, and five homoeopathic dilutions. Proprietary products are preferable for reasons of sterility, e.g. Weleda Euphrasia Eye Drops.

2.7 Oral Candidiasis

Thrush is relatively common in infants. Creamy white stipples or patches of exudate indicate the yeast infection. A tried and tested phytomedicine, the efficacy of which has been substantiated in recent trials, is **tincture of myrrh (Tinctura Myrrhae)**. It is applied with the aid of a cotton-wool tip, undiluted for small areas and diluted 1:1 with boiled water or, even better, chamomile tea, for larger areas.

A mouthwash consisting of a 10% decoction of bilberries (Myrtilli fructus) has also proved effective.

2.8 Scabies and Head Lice

In spite of improved hygienic conditions, children are still quite frequently infested with **itch mite** and **head lice**.

The **itch mite** may cause eczema, inflammatory and purulent lesions. The mites can usually be seen as black dots in the skin. **Peru balsam** has proved its value as a phytotherapeutic antiparasitic. It is applied in ointment form or as a shaking mixture. Follow-up treatment for skin reactions may consist in washing with aqueous extracts of Equisetum herb combined 2:1 with chamomile flowers. The method of preparation is as follows: Add 100 g of Equiseti herba conc. to 2 litres of boiling water and keep on a low flame for 10 minutes; add 50 g of Matricariae flos, turn off the heat and leave to stand for 10 minutes before straining. Wash the area up to five times a day with this extract/infusion.

The **house dust mite**, a fairly ubiquitous parasite, evokes allergic reactions in the skin and respiratory tract. The first step is to prevent exposure, but in the majority of cases the prescription of antiallergic drugs will be unavoidable.

Head lice, mainly seen in schoolchildren, cause pruritus, reddening of the scalp and nits (ova) fixed to the hair shafts. The phytotherapeutic alternative to the generally used organochloride pesticides (e.g. γ-HCH) are pyrethrum extracts made from the flowers of the African *Chrysanthemum cinerarii* (Trev.) Vis. A number of preparations are on the market, among them Goldgeist forte liquidum and Jacutin®-N-Lösung (lotion).

Two preparations which have, quite rightly, fallen into desuetude are Sabadilla vinegar (Acetum Sabadillae), produced from sabadilla seeds by pharmacists, and acetic tincture of sabadilla (Tinctura Sabadillae acetosa). Both have effective antiparasitic properties but their active constituents are highly toxic steroid alkaloids.

2.9 External Applications for Respiratory Tract Diseases

Ointments, baths and **inhalations** have proved highly efficacious volatile oil applications in paediatrics as they are well tolerated (for proprietary products, see p. 32). Fig. 7 gives an overview of the different applications. Despite the conventional view that there is no specific treatment for "common" respiratory tract infections, volatile oils may be said to be extremely useful natural substances for adjuvant treatment of "common" respiratory infections and the "common" cold. Efficacy has been demonstrated in a number of clinical trials, [35] especially in breast-fed infants, who feed better once the nasal passages have cleared. One advantage is that volatile oils are absorbed via the skin as well as by inhalation, so that the gastrointestinal tract is not directly affected. Details are given in handbooks [40, 41] and a number of publications. [36−39]

Rubbing ointments containing volatile oils (see p. 31 and 32) into the chest and back has proved particularly efficacious with infants and young children. The risk of undesirable bronchospasms [42, 43] is extremely low with percutaneous application; they do occur now and then due to inhalation overdosage (> 15 g of ointment per inhalation dose).

Ointments containing menthol and/or camphor must not be applied directly to the inside of the nose, nor in the immediate vicinity of the nose. It is generally known that wrong use of menthol-containing medicines can cause the "Kratschmer" reflex of apnoea and instant collapse, [39] and manufacturers have to some extent responded by producing separate products suitable for babies (e.g. Pinimenthol®-S-Salbe [ointment]), but it is important to draw attention to this potential side effect. This is where pharmacists have an important role to play in providing essential information. Not more than a **hand's breadth** of ointments containing menthol should be rubbed into back and chest.

The Commission E Monographs (Chapter 5) list the following volatile oils or preparations made with them:

- Camphora   (a),
- Eucalypti aetheroleum and
  Eucalypti folium   (b),
- Menthae arvensis and Menthae
  piperitae aetheroleum   (c),
- Piceae turiones recentes   (d),
- Pini aetheroleum   (e),
- Terebinthinae aetheroleum
  rectificatum   (f)

on the following indications:
- catarrhal conditions
  of respiratory tract   (a),
- respiratory tract infections   (b),
- upper respiratory tract catarrh   (c),
- respiratory tract catarrh   (d),
- catarrhal conditions of upper and
  lower respiratory tract   (e),
- chronic diseases of bronchi
  with increased mucus   (f).

Good results have been obtained with the NRF 4.3 formulation **"Inhalatio composita"**, especially for coryza and nasal catarrh:

Eucalyptus oil	4.5 g
Pumilio pine oil	4.5 g
Peppermint oil	1.0 g

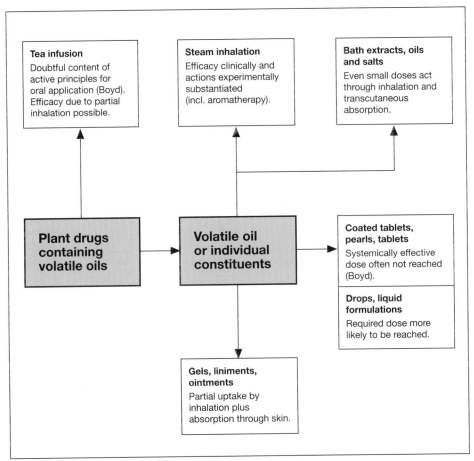

Fig. 7. Overview of potential applications of volatile oils and preparations containing them

For inhalations, add not more than **3 to 5 drops** of the mixture to 1 litre of hot water.

It is important to keep the water sufficiently hot for some time, as adequate amounts of the volatile oil will only evaporate at temperatures above 90 °C, especially if sesquiterpene compounds (e.g. chamazulene) are involved.

Only the steam inhalation recommended by Römmelt et al. [95] would ensure water temperatures of not less than 90 °C. It involves keeping the vessel containing the hot water and volatile oil on a hot plate.

The plastic inhalers that are now available are a compromise solution, for the mask allows the vapour to reach the respiratory tract directly. Rapid cooling of the water may be prevented by using insulated systems (e.g. Pinimenthol® Thermo-Inhalator, Bronchoforton® Inhalator). With these, the water temperature is still at about 75 °C after 10 minutes. If patients (especially children) find the inhalation too hot at first, it is possible to vary the distance between nose and inhaler orifice. At a distance of 10 cm the steam has cooled to about 50 °C.

If the inhaler does not have insulation (e.g. Kamillosan® Inhalator) it is best to use half the amount of boiling water at first, adding the rest after about 5 minutes. Scientific information on the inhalation of volatile oils and the chemical data of individual volatile oil constituents may be found in Römmelt et al. [95] Inhalation using ultrasound vaporizers has proved effective in paediatrics. **It is important to note the contraindications given in the Monographs (Chapter 5).**

Comment. Inhalations have been included in Chapter 2, "Phytopharmaceutic Preparations for **External** Use", for reasons connected with teaching practice. It is, of course, internationally accepted that inhalations rate as internal applications. A discussion of oral exhibition of phytopharmaceutical drugs containing volatile oils to treat respiratory conditions follows immediately, at the beginning of Chapter 3.

2.9.1 Proprietary Products

Bronchoforton® Kinderbalsam (balsam for children) or Bronchofortan® Kinderkombi (paediatric comb.), Expectal® Balsam, Liniplant® Inhalat, Makatussin Balsam mild, Monapax Hustenbalsam (cough balsam), Pertussin® Hustenbalsam, Pinimenthol®-Bad, -Gel, -Liquidum, -Salbe (ointment) (specially for infants), Rhinotussal®-S-Balsam, Soledum®-Balsam, Tumarol-Balsam® sine mentholo, stas® Salbe mild, Thymipin®-Balsam, Babix-Inhalat N.

Monographs

Eucalyptus oil *Ger. P.* 10 (Eucalypti aetheroleum), Peppermint oil *Ger. P.* 10 (Menthae piperitae aetheroleum), Pine needle oil *Ger. P.* 10 (Piceae aetheroleum).

Chapter 3

Phytomedicines for Internal Use in Paediatrics

3.1 Respiratory Tract Diseases

3.1.1 Upper Respiratory Tract Catarrh

Inhalation of volatile oils or preparations containing them, or the use of nebulizers, are the method of choice when treating upper respiratory tract catarrhs in children (see p. 30, 31 and 40).

Other methods of application can complement and enhance the treatment strategy, especially for schoolchildren. They include gargling with aqueous extracts and the taking of medicinal teas, expressed juices and syrups.

Inflammation of the oral and pharyngeal mucosa may be treated by gargling with extracts of **sage leaves, Salviae folium** (botanical name *Salvia officinalis* L.), according to the Commission E Monograph.

The following are recommended for gargling and rinsing:

- Pour ca. 150 ml of boiling water on to 2.5 g (= 1 teaspoonful) of minced sage leaves, leave to infuse for 10 minutes and strain. The lukewarm extract may be used immediately as a gargle. Use 2 or 3 times daily.

- 1 or 2 drops of the volatile sage oil to 100 ml of water.
- 5 g (1 teaspoonful) of the ethanolic extract (tincture) to 1 glass of water.

Gargling with Salviathymol® (10 drops to 1/2 glass of water) has also proved effective.

Dryness of mouth and throat are ameliorated by sucking sage or Iceland moss lozenges (for proprietary products, see p. 40). This measure is especially indicated if the air is dry indoors (central heating).

Pharmacists must take care to dispense leaves of *Salvia officinalis*, also known as "Dalmatian sage" and not to be confused with "Greek sage" (botanical name *Salvia triloba* L. Fil.) or "Spanish sage" (botanical name *Salvia lavandulifolia L.*) There are as yet no Commission E Monographs for the latter two.

Another useful drug for respiratory tract catarrh and inflammatory changes of the oral and pharyngeal mucosa listed by Commission E is **ribwort plantain, Plantaginis lanceolatae herba** (botanical name *Plantago lanceolata* L.). In popular medicine this has been mainly used for coughs. Preparations available are:

- Infusion (3−6 g of the dried plant drug as mean daily dose)
- fresh plant extract (for proprietary products, see p. 40)

- plantain syrup (for proprietary products, see p. 40) (very popular with children)

The **quality requirements** for plantain given below are intended to illustrate the pharmacist's functions in a real and topical example.

Pharmacists must note the proportion of leaf stalks and flowering stems, which should not exceed 1 per cent (note: this is not stated in *Ger. P.* 10, but according to Holz [44] the figure should be as low as possible). Holz also states that the proportion of dark coloured leaves should be as low as possible. Dark coloration indicates decomposition of the iridoid glycosides (including 0.3−2.7% of aucubin, depending on provenance and production conditions) with their antibacterial activity. The aglycone aucubigenin is unstable and polymerizes to form dark brown compounds without antibacterial activity.

Poor quality plant materials, generally collected in the wild, are to be replaced by intensified commercial production of *Plantago lanceolata*. In Holland, work has been in progress for some time to develop a variety of high pharmaceutical quality.

Another plant drug that is less well known but can be recommended for paediatric use because it is well tolerated is downy **hemp-nettle**, **Galeopsidis herba** (botanical name: *Galeopsis segetum* Necker). Infusions are used (6 g of the dried plant drug as mean daily dose). Personal experience has shown that children will happily take the following tea mixture:

Galeopsidis herba conc.	60.0 g
Serpylli herba conc.	40.0 g

Dosage: A cupful several times daily, always using 1 tablespoonful of the tea mixture and 150 ml of boiling water; 1 teaspoonful for the mixture is sufficient for infants.

The Commission E Monograph gives "mild respiratory tract catarrh" as the indication for downy hemp-nettle.

According to the available scientific data, **senega root**, **Polygalae radix** (botanical name *Polygala senega* L. and closely related species) is certainly suitable for treating upper respiratory tract catarrhs, but it is not really suitable for paediatric use. It has the undesirable side effect of gastrointestinal irritation (see Monograph in the appendix).

3.1.2 Unproductive Cough

Treatment for **cough** in paediatrics should be directed to the **symptoms** of **acute tracheobronchitis** rather than **chronic bronchitis**.

The "cough phytomedicines" given below are **not antitussives** in the strict pharmacological sense, even if those containing mucilage may be said to have some "antitussive activity". They are primarily **expectorants**. For prescriptions, and above all for self-medication and when making over-the-counter recommendations in the pharmacy, distinction should/must be made between

- **unproductive cough** and
- **cough producing viscous mucus** (productive cough) difficult to cough up.

With **unproductive cough**, useful medicinal actions would be a) reduction or suppression of the cough reflex in the brain stem and b) blocking sensitive receptors ("cough receptors" in the bronchial tract). Mucilages address the second of these, reducing hypersensitivity of cough receptors in the upper respiratory tract. **Codeine** and **noscapine** act as cough suppressants. Noscapine does not have the side effects seen with codeine and is therefore the antitussive to be prescribed instead of codeine in paediatrics.

Plant mucilages (mucilaginosa) primarily relieve coughs by covering the inflamed mucosa with a kind of protective layer, preventing exogenic irritants (e.g. dust) from reaching the mechano- or chemoreceptors. A second hypothesis for their action which is still in dispute suggests reflex relief of cough by reducing nervus vagus sensitivity. Be that as it may, the efficacy of some mucilaginosa is beyond dispute, and in paediatrics they are preferable to many of the widely advertised "chemical wonder drugs".

Commission E gave "irritation of oral and pharyngeal mucosa in conjunction with unproductive, dry cough" as the indication for **marshmallow root, Althaeae radix** (botanical name *Althaea officinalis* L.). The Monograph lists the following actions, based on current scientific knowledge: "demulcent and emollient, inhibition of mucociliar activity, with increased phagocytosis". **Sirupus Althaeae** is a particularly suitable formulation in paediatrics, as children generally like it. The single dose, which may be repeated several times daily, is 2−8 ml (small teaspoonful to 2 tablespoonfuls) according to age. Marshmallow syrup may be prescribed as a generic or proprietary preparation (see p. 40).

Care must be taken to use cold water when making marshmallow root tea (cold maceration), extracting 1 tablespoonful of minced roots for 2 or 3 hours in 200 ml of cold water. Following the extraction, the liquid is strained off and briefly brought to the boil to kill any microbes present.

Another herbal medicine with the same indication is **Iceland moss, Lichen islandicus** (botanical name *Cetraria islandica* L.). A positive "side effect" – the complexity of phytomedicines has been briefly discussed in Chapter 1 – is the appetite-stimulating effect of aqueous Lichen islandicus. This complementary effect and a weak antimicrobial action make Iceland moss particularly well suited to paediatrics. Clinical studies are in progress.

Iceland moss is entirely collected in the wild and tends to grow in company with other shrubby lichens, and pharmacists as "guardians of quality" must check the plant drug carefully for identity and purity. Following the Chernobyl incident it has been difficult to obtain marketable quality material with less than 600 Bq berilium from Scandinavian countries. Imports from other countries, e.g. Canada, are radiation-free but rarely seen on the market. The situation has improved since 1994.

Monographs for plant drugs to use for nonproductive cough are **mallow flowers and leaves, Malvae flos and Malvae folium** (botanical name *Malva sylvestris* L. and *Malva neglecta* Wallroth). The quality of mallow flowers tends to be poor, but mallow leaves are usually of acceptable quality.

A plant drug that serves both as a basic remedy and a colorant are **mullein flowers, Verbasci flos** (botanical names *Verbascum densiflorum* Bertoline and/ or *Verbascum phlomoides* L.). Infants and young children will happily take teas made with mullein flowers (3−4 g of the dried drug per cup). The method is as follows: To 1 tablespoon of minced mullein flowers add about 200 ml of boiling water and leave to infuse for 15 minutes. Sweeten with honey and serve between meals.

The commercial quality of mullein flowers varies a great deal. Flowers showing dark discoloration must be rejected. Store Verbasci flos in a dry place, also at home.

3.1.3 Cough with Viscid Expectoration (Productive Cough)

Viscid secretions are noticeable from the rattling sound of the cough. Secretolytic and/or secretomotoric agents will be needed to liquefy the viscid mucus and/or get it moving through ciliary action. **Saponin-containing phytomedicines** generally have both those principles of action. Stimulation of ciliary motion triggered by a reflex mechanism from the stomach, via vagus stimulation, is the primary action. Sputum viscosity decreases, not due to degradation of mucopolysaccharides, as with the mucolytics ambroxol and bromhexine, but probably because the systemically absorbed saponins reduce the surface tension of the sputum. The action is therefore not the same as that of synthetic mucolytics. Increased activity of ciliary epithelium as an expectorant action has been experimentally established for a number of saponin drugs. [45, 46]

The most widely known saponin cough medicament is **liquorice root, Liquiritiae radix** (botanical name *Glycyrrhiza glabra* L.), though for lack of clinical trials the Commission E Monograph only gives "Catarrhal conditions of upper respiratory tract and gastric/duodenal ulcer" as indications. The Monograph does, however, explicitly state that secretolytic and expectorant actions have been demonstrated in animal experiments. Liquorice root is usually part of cough tea mixtures such as Species pectorales *Ger. P.* 6:

Althaeae radix conc.	8 parts
Liquiritiae radix conc.	4 parts

Farfarae folium conc.	4 parts
Verbasci flos conc.	2 parts
Anisi fructus tot.	2 parts

Dosage: a cupful several times daily, made with 1 tablespoonful of the mixture. Half the dose is recommended for infants.

A standard mixture for "cough tea" and for catarrhal conditions of the upper respiratory tract recommended by Commission E is the following:
Recipe:

Liquiritiae radix conc.	50.0 g
Primulae radix conc.	10.0 g
Althaeae radix conc.	30.0 g
Anisi fructus tot.	10.0 g

Signa: Species pectorales
Dosis: Up to 5 cups daily, made as an infusion using 1 teaspoonful of the mixture, to be taken as hot as possible.

Inspissated liquorice juice, Succus Liquiritiae, is widely used especially in paediatrics. The recommended daily dose is 0.5 – 1.0 g. The formula for a popular "liquorice cough mixture for children" is the following:

Succus Liquiritiae	10.0 g
Tinctura Aurantii	2.0 g
Liquor Ammonii anisatus	5.0 g
Sirupus Rubi Idaei	ad 100.0 g

Dosage: 1 teaspoonful up to 5 times daily, preferably dissolved in milk. (Because of the taste, it may be advisable to reduce the Succus Liquiritiae to 5.0 g for young children. It is also possible to replace the raspberry syrup with Sirupus simplex.)

The *German Pharmacopoeia* 10 requires the unpeeled root, which may be from China, Spain, the South of France or Italy. However, the peeled Russian liquorice root has much better taste and is therefore more suitable for paediatric use.

It is stated in the Monograph that if used for some time and in relatively high doses (especially if the concentration of the triterpene saponin glycyrrhizin is relatively high) **mineralocorticoid effects** such as sodium and water retention, potassium loss, hypertension, oedema and hypokalaemia develop. Note should be taken of this. With short-term treatment given for cough, especially if using Liquiritiae radix, these mineralocorticoid effects do **not** develop. Quite logically, therefore, it says that there are no known side effects, which is true if used according to the rules, when so far no side effects have been reported.*

Ivy leaves, **Hederae helicis folium** (botanical name *Hedera helix* L.), for which a Monograph also exists, are not suitable for paediatric use as teas infused at home. The mean daily dose of 0.3 g of the drug is only too easily exceeded, and tea preparations tend to contain variable saponin mixtures (e.g. bisdesmoside B and C, or monodesmoside α- and β-hederine). Use of a standardized ivy leaf extract, on the other hand, has proved very useful in paediatrics. The extract is standardized for a specific spasmolytic activity (1 g of the extract is equivalent to 10 mg of papaverine) and being in liquid form it is easy to keep the dose accurate (= Prospan®). Since 1995 standardization is phytochemical as well as biological.

Oxlip and cowslip flowers and roots, **Primulae flos and Primulae radix** (botanical names *Primula veris* L. and/or *Primula elatior* Hill, L.) are also specially recommended for paediatric use. According to their Monographs both have the same action (secretolytic and expectorant) and indications. According to certain scientific data, however, the flowers are more suitable for paediatric use than the roots. Biochemically this is borne out by the lower saponin content and better organoleptic properties (yellow colour and better taste of cowslip flower tea). If the pharmacist offers the right advice and dispenses good-quality Primulae flos (flowers with calices, as only these contain saponins) he is "doing his part" in two respects in a scientifically orientated strategy for phytotherapy.

The mean daily dose for cowslip flowers is 3 g of the dried plant drug, for the roots only 1 g of the dried plant drug; alternatively 1.5−3.0 g of tincture of cowslip root or 2.5−7.5 g of cowslip or oxlip flower tincture.

Finally there is the **alkaloid-containing drug ipecacuanha (vomiting root)**, **Ipecacuanhae radix** (botanical names *Cephaelis ipecacuanha* [Brot.] Rich, A. and/or *Cephaelis acuminata* Karsten). A Monograph for the indication "cough" is not available and Commission E is not at present planning to produce one. The pharmacodynamics are different from those of the above saponin drugs, yet the indication for cough is approximately the same. Extracts of ipecacuanha root have a powerful secretolytic action, [46] but great care must be taken over dosage, as higher doses will quickly cause vomiting. This emetic effect is due to marked local irritation of the gastric mucosa. Teas of ipecacuanha root must therefore never be used in paediatrics. **Ipecacuanha tincture** (*Ger. P.* 10) is suitable, however, as it is standardized for a specific alkaloid content of not less than 0.19 and not more than 0.21 % and can be given in accurate doses. Depending on the child's age, the single dose is 10 to 30 drops of the tincture given in milk or herb tea. Higher doses of the tincture (more than 2 mg total alkaloid content per single dose) are an extremely useful

---

* In paediatrics, use according to the rules means a daily dose not exceeding 1.0 g of Succus Liquiritiae for a period not exceeding 6 weeks.

emetic in cases of poisoning. Details of this will be given later (p. 64 and 65).

An "aromatic" syrup of vomiting root made to the following formula has also proved its value in paediatrics, though adequate precautions must be taken:

Ipecacuanhae tinctura *Ger. P.* 10 with standardized alkaloid content   10.0 g
Aurantii tinctura or Aromatica
tinctura   1.0 g
Sirupus simplex   ad 100.0 g

Dosage: 1 teaspoonful 3 times daily for infants from 1 year of age. **Do not give more than 1 teaspoonful per dose!** (See also under 3.7.)

3.1.4 Whooping Cough

It is important to remember that **pertussis** is an acute infectious disease of the respiratory tract. It is one of the most life-threatening respiratory diseases in early infancy. The characteristic feature are repeated, severe bouts of coughing. The pathogen, *Bordetella pertussis*, produces a toxin that may cause necrosis and ulceration in the bronchial tract, resulting in the well-known coughing attacks in the paroxysmal stage. According to Prof. Stehr from the University Hospital for Children in Erlangen, Germany, about 100,000 children a year contract whooping cough in the Federal Republic (1993).

Phytomedicines will merely reduce the severity of the paroxysmal attacks. They can also prevent congestion of the clear, viscid mucus. Phytotherapy cannot be used to treat the causes. The conventional medical view is that because of the highly infectious nature of the condition, antibiotics need to be given for an extended period, at every stage, despite the fact that the clinical symptoms at the paroxysmal stage will not respond to antibiotics.

Adjuvant treatment may include the following:

Ivy leaves, **Hederae helicis folium**, though it is important to use only standardized extracts. Prospan® suppositories have proved particularly useful, also Children's Linctus.

Another "whooping cough drug" is **sundew**, **Droserae herba** (botanical names *Drosera rotundifolia* L., *Drosera ramentacea* Burch ex Harv. et Sond., *Drosera longifolia* L. and *Drosera intermedia* Hayne). The listing of several species reflects the current supply situation, with the originally used *Drosera rotundifolia* now a protected plant and no longer available. Comparative analysis of the above species showed them to be equal as far as their main active principles were concerned (e.g. naphthoquinone derivatives).[48] The Commission E Monograph lists "paroxysmal and unproductive cough" under Indications and "bronchospasmolytic, antitussive" under Actions. Ethanolic extracts are more effective, especially if combined with a small number of other agents as standardized fluidextracts. The proprietary preparations Pertussin® forte is a well established, effective adjuvant in the treatment of pertussis and chronic laryngitis. Interestingly enough, Prof. of Medicine Ernst Fischer at Strasbourg University reported on good clinical results with Pertussin syrup as early as 1898.[49]

The most important other substance in the above-mentioned proprietary preparations is **thyme**, **Thymi herba** (botanical names *Thymus vulgaris* and *Thymus zygis* L.). The Commission E Monograph lists "symptoms of bronchitis and **whooping cough**, upper respiratory catarrh" under Indications and "bronchospasmolytic, expectorant, antibacterial" under Actions. Thyme tea (about 150 ml of boiling water poured over 1−2 g of the dried plant drug and left to infuse for about 10 minutes) taken several times a day should be sufficient for the treatment of upper respiratory catarrh, but for adjuvant treatment of pertussis it is necessary to use an ethanolic extract, preferably Thymi extractum fluidum *Ger. P.* 10. Ethanolic extracts generally contain adequate amounts of volatile oils, including the isomeric monoterpenes thymol and carvacrol. Thymol with its phenol coefficient of 20 is a natural product with good disinfectant properties. Thyme oil therefore heads the list of volatile oils with antibacterial properties,[36] with the thymol content an important quality criterion for all thyme preparations.

The "thyme taste", generally popular with children, is another good reason for including thyme in compound preparations. Cough syrups smelling and tasting of thyme are happily taken even by young children.

A standard combination of sundew herb and thyme herb also has Commission E approval (Federal Gazette No. 67, 4 Apr 1992).

In conclusion, a **useful tea mixture** for the symptomatic treatment of paroxysmal and whooping cough :

Thymi herba conc.	40.0 g
Droserae herba conc.	40.0 g
Anisi fructus tot.	15.0 g
Verbasci flos conc.	5.0 g

Dosage: 1 cupful, made by infusing 1 tablespoonful of the mixture in 150 ml of boiling water, several times daily.

A tried and tested fluid formulation is the following:
Recipe:

Tinctura Droserae	5.0 g
Extractum Thymi fluidum	ad 20.0 g

Dosage: 20−30 drops several times daily, in milk.

3.1.5 Rhinitis

To conclude the section on Respiratory Tract Diseases brief reference shall be made to "aromatherapy" to treat **rhinitis**. For details, see section 2.9, pages 30 and 31. Treatment is merely symptomatic, but it does considerably reduce the time the disease takes and because of the antibacterial action of the above-mentioned volatile oils also makes a major contribution in preventing superinfection. A useful method is to put a few drops of mint oil on a handkerchief and "sniff" this. Recent clinical trials have yielded scientific proof of efficacy for mint oil in the treatment of rhinitis.

3.1.6 Sinusitis

Acute sinusitis, often the consequence of an earlier episode that was not fully overcome or wrongly treated, can be successfully treated by inhalation of volatile oils with antibacterial and antiinflammatory activities. The first to be considered is "chamomile steam inhalation". Care must be taken to see that the steam phase contains adequate amounts of the volatile chamomile oil; this is achieved by using 10−20 ml of a standardized proprietary chamomile preparation. With sinusitis it is particularly important to use the correct method of inhalation (see p. 31 and 32).

Chronic sinusitis sometimes requires surgical treatment.[27] A number of individual successes achieved by nasal irrigation with the following solution

Tinctura Calendulae (mother tincture)	20.0 g
Tinctura Echinaceae (mother tincture)	1.0 g
physiological saline	ad 100.0 g

3 times daily, still require clinical confirmation. This nasal irrigation should as a

rule only be used with schoolchildren and young people.

Chronic sinusitis generally reflects recurrent infectious conditions,[70] and should therefore not be treated without medical supervision. The causal factors have to be taken into account, and apart from drops to reduce swelling, antibiotics are usually required. Concurrent use of a herbal secretolytic (e.g. Sinupret® liquid) has, however, proved highly efficacious.

3.1.7 Proprietary Products

a) **Upper respiratory catarrh**
Salviathymol® liquidum, Isla-Moos® lozenges, Kneipp® Spitzwegerich (ribwort plantain) fresh plant extract, Dr med. Otto Greither Spitzwegerichsaft (ribwort plantain juice), Denosol® mild spray

b) **Cough**
Sirupus Althaeae *Ger. P.* 6, Liquiritiae extractum fluidum *Ger. P.* 10, Succus Liquiritiae depuratus *Ger. P.* 6, Ipecacuanhae extractum and tinctura *Ger. P.* 10 Biotuss®cough syrup for children (= Sirupus Althaeae plus thyme fluidextract and Drosera 2x), Eupatal® drops and syrup, Hustagil® cough syrup, Makatussin® drops and linctus, Melrosum® syrup, Kneipp® thyme herbal syrup, Pertussin® cough syrup, Thymipin® cough drops, etc.

Whooping cough
Drosithyn® Bürger drops, Hustagil® Thymiantropfen (thyme drops) forte, Prospan® drops and suppositories, Pertussin® cough drops, Thymipin® forte drops

c) **Rhinitis**
Liniplant® inhalation, Pumilen® nose drops and inhalation, Denosol® mild spray for colds, Emser Nasensalbe (nasal ointment)

d) **Sinusitis**
Kamillosan® drops, Sinupret® drops, Oleum Thymi *Ger. P.* 6 for inhalation.

3.2 Colds

(excluding rhinitis, respiratory catarrh, cough, etc. – see p. 39 ff.)

Phytotherapy given in addition to physical (e.g. wet compresses around the lower legs for pyrexia) and dietetic measures (e.g. a light but palatable diet) can often be a highly useful complementary strategy in the treatment of common cold. For both self-medication and home nursing without medical advice it is important to note that if the condition persists, medical advice must be sought and a differential diagnosis made. Above all it is necessary to exclude "genuine" influenza, though this is less common in children and young people, infectious mononucleosis, bacterial infection (e.g. streptococcal throat, *Haemophilus influenzae*, etc.) and pseudovirus infection (e.g. psittacosis, mycoplasmal pneumonia, etc.). It is also important to know that the phytopharmaceutic drugs mentioned below have no effect on rhinoviruses (RNA viruses of the Picornaviridae family) or coronaviruses (RNA viruses of the Coronaviridae family). Virostatic activities so far established for natural substances or plant extracts essentially relate only to herpes viruses. Personal studies with propolis extracts and individual propolis constituents are in progress and virostatic activity has been established.

Phytotherapy may be used to reduce or ameliorate general symptoms such as

- reduced general condition (loss of appetite, malaise)
- pain in limbs and muscles
- headache
- inflammatory changes in the respiratory tract
- pyrexia

Proper advice consists in first of all suggesting measures not involving medication:

- bed rest
- plenty of hot liquids, preferably herbal teas made with fruits, or juices (e.g. elderberry or bilberry)
- cool compresses applied to the throat and lower legs for pyrexia
- ensure air is not dry in the sick-room (evaporation of water, etc.)

3.2.1 Antipyretic Herbal Preparations

Antipyretic herbal medicines include **willow bark**, **Salicis cortex** (botanical names *Salix alba* L. and *Salix fragilis* L.) with total salicin content not less than 1%. The Commission E Monograph lists "febrile conditions, rheumatic complaints, headache" under Indications and "antipyretic, antiinflammatory and analgesic" under Actions. The mean daily adult dose is given as 60−120 mg of total salicin; this is equivalent to 6−12 g of the dried plant drug. Paediatric doses are 15 mg of total salicin/kg of body weight from the age of 3 months onwards. Children will often refuse to take **willow bark tea** because of the taste but are usually happy to accept it in a **mixture**. The Commission E Monograph explicitly states: "Combination with diaphoretic herbal preparations may be very effective".

An effective **"influenza tea"** for children may be formulated as follows:
Salicis cortex conc. (antipyretic)   30.0 g
Tiliae flos conc. (diaphoretic)   40.0 g
Spiraeae flos conc. (antipyretic, diaphoretic)   10.0 g
Matricariae flos tot. (antiinflammatory, spasmolytic)   10.0 g
Aurantii pericarpium conc. (appetite stimulating, flavour improver)   10.0 g
Dosage: 1 cupful 3−4 times daily, made as an infusion using 1 tablespoonful of the mixture, left to infuse for about 10 minutes.

Proprietary preparations (see p. 45) based on standardized willow bark extracts are particularly useful as it is possible to use exact dosage.

Two other **antipyretic** herbal drugs are **meadowsweet flowers and herb**, Spiraeae flos and Spiraeae herba (botanical name *Filipendula ulmaria* Maximowicz, L.). The flowers have greater medicinal value, added to which is their pleasant scent and taste. The Commission E Monograph lists "colds" under Indications; the mean daily dose is 2−3 g of the flowers or 4−6 g of the herb, used as an infusion. For paediatric use, use 1 teaspoonful of meadowsweet flowers or 1 tablespoonful of the herb to a cup, up to 4 times daily.

3.2 Diaphoretic Herbal Preparations

The most important are **lime blossom**, Tiliae flos, and **elder flower**, Sambuci flos. For **lime blossom** (botanical names *Tilia cordata* Miller and *Tilia platyphyllos* Scopoli), recent clinical and experimental work has been done to establish efficacy and activity. [50] Before this was published, Commission E had already approved the following indications: "Adjuvant treatment of colds, mucosal irritation in mouth and throat and the dry cough associated with this". Children like a mixture of

Tiliae flos conc.	80.0 g
Menthae piperitae folium conc.	20.0 g

Dosage: 1 cupful of the tea made with 1 tablespoonful of the mixture infused for 10 minutes, taken as hot as possible.

Note should be taken that **lime flowers** are sometimes **substituted** with other species. Flowers of *Tilia tomentosa* Moench (syn. *Tilia argentea* DC = silver lime) and *Tilia* x *euchlora* Koch, C. are the most commonly found substitute on the market. [51] Both are popular ornamental trees also grown in avenues. The bracts and leaves of silver lime are densely hairy compared to those of small and large leaved limes. Substitution is therefore recognizable from the hairy bracts (which are part of the inflorescence and therefore part of the plant drug) and the unpleasant, repulsive odour and taste of the aqueous extract.

The Commission E Monograph for **elder flower**, Sambuci flos (botanical name *Sambucus nigra* L.), lists "colds" under Indications and "**diaphoretic**; increases bronchial secretion" under Actions. The mean daily dose of 10−15 g of the dried plant drug seems rather high;

work is in progress to check this. In paediatric practice, the recommended maximum daily dose is 3 tablespoonfuls of elder flowers (infusion).

Below is a formula for **Species diaphoreticae, specially for children**:

Tiliae flos conc.	70.0 g
Spiraeae flos conc.	10.0 g
Menthae piperitae folium conc.	15.0 g
Aurantii pericarpium conc.	5.0 g

Dosage: Prior to taking physical measures to induce sweating, 1 cup to be taken as hot as possible. Use 1 tablespoonful of the mixture to 150 ml of boiling water and leave to infuse to 10 minutes.

Improvement in the poor general condition, generally combined with **loss of appetite** and **malaise**, should be the second phytotherapeutic measure in the treatment of colds, though depending on the case it may also be the first.

3.2.3 Aperitive Herbal Preparations

The most important **appetite-stimulating drugs** currently included in the Commission E list on the indications "Loss of appetite and indigestion" and useful in paediatrics are the **aromatic bitters** (Tables 1 and 2). They include wormwood herb (Absinthii herba) in low doses, bitter orange peel (Aurantii pericarpium), sage leaves (Salviae folium) and especially, in paediatrics, sweet flag root (Calami rhizoma) and eagle vine bark (Condurango cortex). They are discussed more fully in the next Chapter (pages 46 and 48).

The following are available from pharmacies and recommended (also in the hope that individual prescriptions made by a physician will come to play a more important role again):

Table 1. Commission E Monographs with the indications loss of appetite, indigestion or dyspeptic symptoms

Bitters (amara)	Centaurii herba, Cichorii herba, Cichorii radix, Cnici benedicti herba, Condurango cortex, Cynarae folium, Gentianae radix, Harpagophyti radix, Taraxaci radix cum herba, Taraxaci herba
Aromatics	Anethi fructus, Anisi fructus, Anisi stellati fructus, Cardamomi fructus, Coriandri fructus, Curcumae longae rhizoma, Curcumae xanthorrhizae rhizoma, Foeniculi fructus, Galangae rhizoma, Juniperi fructus, Zingiberis rhizoma
Aromatic bitters	Absinthii herba, Aurantii pericarpium, Salviae folium
Volatile sulphur compounds	Allii cepae bulbus, Raphani sativi radix
Flavonoids	Cardui mariae fructus, Helichrysi flos, flower pollen

Aurantii tinctura   *Ger. P.* 10
Dosage: 30−50 drops before meals.
Cinchonae tinctura composita *Ger. P.* 10
Dosage: 20−30 drops before meals.
Tinctura aromatica   *Ger. P.* 6
Dosage: 30−40 drops before meals.
Tinctura calami   *Ger. P.* 6
Dosage: 30−50 drops before meals.
Vinum chinae   *Ger. P.* 6
Dosage: 1 tablespoonful before meals.
Vinum condurango   *Ger. P.* 6
Dosage: 1 or 2 tablespoonfuls before meals.
All the above ethanolic extracts are best taken in fruit juice or herbal tea.

With medicinal wines, which contain approx. 16 vol.% of alcohol, it is of course important to use a dosage suitable for children. This also applies to many proprietary roborants, by the way. Infants do not produce alcohol dehydrogenase. Alcoholic preparations can therefore only be given from the 13th month onwards as a rule.

3.2.4 Immunomodulators formerly Immunostimulators

The third measure frequently taken by paediatricians is to **increase resistance** or restore it to normal. A chill (wet feet, wet clothing, no head covering) frequently reduces the immune defences. Treatment with herbal "immunostimulants", [52] now known as "immunomodulators" will only serve a purpose if applied at the first signs of a cold, or even prophylactically – and then for a short period only. [52] A plant that has been thoroughly investigated, [53] even if the mechanism of action at the molecular level is not yet known, is the **herb of coneflower**, Echinaceae purpureae herba (botanical name *Echinacea purpurea* Moench, L.). The Commission E Monograph lists under Indications: "Adjuvant treatment of recurrent infections in the respiratory and lower urinary tracts". It is interesting to see the details given as to Actions: "In humans

Table 2. Commission E Monographs with indications other than loss of appetite and dyspeptic symptoms

Dyspeptic symptoms, mild exocrine pancreatic insufficiency	Harunganae madagascariensis cortex et folium
Functional epigastric symptoms (nervous stomach, Roehmheld's gastrocardial syndrome, meteorism, intestinal problems of nervous origin)	Lavandulae flos
Mucilage for gastritis and enteritis	Lini semen
Gastric and duodenal ulcers	Liquiritiae radix
Gastrointestinal spasms and inflammatory conditions of the gastrointestinal tract	Matricariae flos
Functional gastrointestinal complaints	Melissae folium
Functional disorders of stomach, intestines and gall-bladder, meteorism	Menthae arvensis aetheroleum (= mint oil)
Spasms in upper gastrointestinal tract and bile ducts	Menthae piperitae aetheroleum (= peppermint oil)
Spasms in gastrointestinal region, gall bladder and bile ducts	Menthae piperitae folium
Low-dose tannins for gastritis and enteritis	Rhei radix
Indigestion, prevention of travel sickness	Zingiberis rhizoma

and animals, Echinacea preparations given parenterally and/or orally have shown **immunobiological activity**. Among other things they elevate the white cell and splenic cell count, activate the phagocytic activity of human macrophages and act as pyrogens." This refers only to the species *Echinacea purpurea*, which is used in relatively few proprietaries (see p. 45). Efficacy differs markedly with oral and parenteral exhibition.

Commission E has not yet felt in a position to make similar statements relating to *Echinacea angustifolia*. According to the team working with Prof. Wagner in Munich [54] and on the basis of a recent double blind trial, *Echinacea angustifolia* and *Echinacea pallida* clearly also rank as a herbal immunostimulants. It is a constituent of most currently available immunostimulants, some of which have come out very well in clinical trials. Unfortunately it is only rarely stated if the proprietary product used in such a trial actually contained *Echinacea angustifolia* or *Echinacea pallida*. Heubl and Bauer [72] have fully reported on confusion between *Echinacea angustifolia* and *Echinacea pallida* and recently also *Parthenium integrifolium*, and on substitution of the latter for *Echinacea purpurea* roots.

In view of recent clinical trials, even without the pharmaceutical problem fully resolved, and of the experimental findings of Prof. Wagner's team [73] we can and must recognize that Echinaceae preparations have clinical efficacy, even if rational treatment is only possible within limits. A number of paediatricians have spoken in highly positive terms to me about the preparations, which lends weight to my opinion, though few other scientific views have been given. [74]

Further immunostimulant medicinal plants are **hemp agrimony (*Eupatorium cannabinum* L.)**, **eupatorium (*Eupatorium perfoliatum* L.)**, **yellow cedar or Arbor vitae (*Thuja occidentalis* L.)** and **pokeweed (*Phytolacca americana* L.)**. They are usually contained in standard compound preparations or used as homoeopathic mother tinctures.

The poll of paediatricians showed that on the basis of almost daily experience each was convinced of the efficacy of "his" herbal immunostimulant, with 4 preparations prescribed by more than one paediatrician (see below). The poll also revealed that little thought was given to molecular mechanisms of action. There was, however, general agreement that the medicament needs to be given at the **onset** of the disease, and then ideally at night and in the mornings and for not more than 4 days if given by mouth. The first dose should be between 40 and 80 drops, depending on age. The majority view is that long-term prophylaxis is not to be recommended, whereas treatment given at intervals has proved effective! This strategy also makes sense theoretically.

3.2.5 Proprietary Products

a) **Pyrexia and pain in extremities**
   Phytodolor® N drops, Salus Schmerzetten® coated tablets
b) **Herbal immunostimulants**
   Echinacea purpurea forte Hervet® drops, Echinacin® Liquidum, Salus® Echinacea drops, Echinatruw® drops, Echinafors Liquidum, Exberitox® N solution and suppositories, Immunopret®, Resplant® capsules and syrup without ethanol, Contramutan® drops, children's linctus and children's suppositories (combination of a number of homoeopathic mother tinctures), Phytolacca mother tincture.

3.3 Diseases of the Gastrointestinal Tract

Diseases or symptoms of the intestinal tract are common in infants, children and young people. Rapid action is generally required, which is why self-medication ranks high in this area. Primarily the conditions are the following:

- Loss or disorder of appetite
- "upset stomach"
- indigestion with meteorism and flatulence
- chronic constipation

3.3.1 Loss of Appetite

Tables 1 and 2 (p. 43 and 44) list all plant drugs for **"loss of appetite, indigestion"** for which monographs exist to date. Below, only those suitable for use in paediatrics will be discussed, plus a few plant drugs for which monographs have not yet been produced.

Children particularly like extracts of bitter orange peel, **Aurantii pericarpium** (botanical name *Citrus aurantium* L., subspecies *amara* Engler). The bitter value of the peel is only 600, but they contain 1–2% of volatile oil with excellent aroma. Bitter orange peel tea, about 2 g (1 teaspoonful to a cup) or, better, 20 drops of bitter orange peel tincture may be given in a cup of peppermint tea before every meal.

Aromatic bitters should definitely be given preference in paediatrics, and that includes **sweet flag**, **Calami rhizoma** (botanical name *Acorus calamus*). The doyen of phytotherapy, Prof. R. F. Weiss, holds sweet flag root in high esteem. In his textbook [1] we read: "The sweet flag has a powerful tonic effect on the stomach, encouraging its secretory activity. It has remarkable powers of stimulating appetite. … Anorexia nervosa and the lack of appetite shown by asthenic, neuropathic young girls appear to respond particularly well to Calamus. Children with **umbilical colic**, and most of all **children with loss of appetite**, or rather with appetite disorders, will very often make a striking recovery if a few drops of Calamus tincture are given regularly before meals. A feature that makes Calamus all the more valuable is that it is not quite so bitter, and is aromatic as well." All we need to add is that one must never use the tetraploid Calamus of Indian or Chinese provenance. The volatile oil of the tetraploid strain contains about 80% of β-asarone. In toxicological studies on rats, this caused malignant tumours in the duodenal region after the 59th week. The diploid *Acorus calamus* strain native to North America and now also cul-

tivated in Europe does not contain β-asarone. The fact that sweet flag root was discredited some years ago was due to lack of sufficient phytochemical information.

Other drugs suitable for the treatment of appetite disorders are **centaury**, **Centaurii herba** (botanical name *Centaurium minus* Moench), **artichoke leaves**, **Cynarae folium** (botanical name *Cynara scolymus* L.) **and eagle vine bark**, **Condurango cortex** (botanical name *Marsdenia condurango* Reichenbach fil.). A relatively low bitter value (800–2000) makes them especially suitable for use in paediatrics.

An appetite-stimulating plant drug that also has general roborant effects recognized by Commission E is **Flower pollen**. Efficacy has been shown specifically for micronized pollen (see proprietary products, p. 53).

A tried and tested formula for achylia, anorexia and "weak stomach" after infections is the following bitter tonic (Amarum tonicum):

Rp Aurantii tinct.   1.0
    Gentianae tinct.   9.0
    Calami tinct.   10.0

M.D.S. 10 drops in 1/2 glass of water before every meal, to be taken in sips. For further formulations, see p. 48 ff.

3.3.2 Gastric Complaints

Gastric upsets of children are quite common in everyday family life and in most cases – unless they keep recurring – can and should be treated from the family medicine chest. The possible causes and symptoms are many and only some of the more relevant are discussed below. Causes may include wrong eating habits (eating too much or too fast, food too cold or too hot, etc.), spoiled food, heavy foods, minor infections, and psychosomatic factors such as school phobia and examination nerves. "Irritable stomach", a condition with purely functional symptoms and no pathological findings, [55] a common cause of gastric upsets in adults, should not be underestimated in children according to some paediatricians.

Symptoms to be mentioned are pain, which tends to move around in the epigastric region, gastric spasms, sensation of fullness, loss of appetite, abnormal taste sensations, nausea, occasionally with vomiting, etc.

Treatment strategy will need to be **dietary** (fasting, light diet, etc.), **psychological** (e.g. a reassuring talk) and/or **phytotherapeutics** as required. In the latter case, plant drugs with the following actions come into consideration:

- spasmolytic
  (to relieve gastric spasms)
- antiinflammatory
  (to reduce irritation of gastric mucosa)
- secretagogue
  (to stimulate secretion of saliva and gastric juices)
- carminative
  (to remove sensation of fullness)
- sedative
  (to calm and soothe generally)
- antimicrobial
  (to inhibit yeast and fungal growth)

The first to be considered are **chamomile flowers**, **Matricariae flos**, preparations with high concentrations of active principles (see p. 53 for proprietary products). Indications for oral use given in the Commission E Monograph are "gastrointestinal spasms and inflammatory diseases of the gastrointestinal tract". For mild complaints, use of "chamomile tea", a tried and tested household remedy, is certainly acceptable, providing it is made with chamomile flowers as defined in the pharmacopoeia. If complaints are more serious and do not improve on chamomile tea, this needs to be reinforced by adding an ethanolic extract (chamomile tincture). The widely available chamomile tea bags are not suitable, especially if purchased anywhere but in a pharmacy, though there are a few exceptions (see p. 53 for proprietary products). Most of the chamomile tea bags sold as non-medicinal drinks do not contain chamomile flowers but chamomile herb, which has extremely low concentrations of volatile oil and flavonoids.

The second plant drug to be considered are **peppermint leaves**, **Menthae piperitae folium** (botanical name *Mentha* x *piperita* L.). The Monograph (see Appendix) lists under Indications: "spasms in area of gastrointestinal tract, gallbladder and bile ducts". It also includes experimentally demonstrated actions that are of interest: "direct spasmolytic effect on smooth musculature of digestive tract, choleretic and carminative".

As already mentioned, not inconsiderable amounts of the volatile oil, and above all of menthol and menthone are transferred to aqueous infusions. [28] It should be added that "peppermint tea" also contains the pharmacologically active "labiate tannins". These include the highly interesting rosemarinic acid and are easily water soluble. Children like to take a tea made with 1 teaspoonful of peppermint leaves and 1/2 teaspoonful of chamomile flowers per cup.

The third plant drug important in paediatrics are **balm leaves**, **Melissae folium** (botanical name *Melissa officinalis* L.). According to the Commission E Monograph, balm leaves may be used on the following indications:

"Functional gastrointestinal disorders, problems going to sleep that are nervous in origin". Here again the water-soluble "labiate tannins" no doubt play a considerable role, due to stimulation of gastric juice and bile production, whilst the concentration of volatile oil would be negligible compared to distilled balm preparations. To make an efficacious tea, 1 tablespoonful of the minced dried plant drug is needed, even for paediatric use, and the tea must be left, covered, to infuse for 15 minutes.

Stomach Tea

The following pleasant-tasting herbal tea mixture is currently being tested for efficacy in the treatment of "minor gastric complaints":

Maricariae flos conc.	50.0 g
Menthae piperitae folium conc.	30.0 g
Melissae folium conc.	15.0 g
Calami rhizoma conc.	5.0 g

Dosage: 3 to 5 cups daily as required, using a heaped teaspoonful to a tablespoonful of the mixture to infuse.

Prof. R. F. Weiss reports good results with the following stomach tea mixture:
Rp Foeniculi fruct. cont.
    Menthae piperitae fol. conc.
    Melissae fol. conc.
    Calami rhizoma conc.   aa 20.0 g
M f. spec. stomachicae
1 teaspoonful to 1 cup of boiling water, leave to infuse for 10 minutes. Drink warm, in sips, 2–3 times daily.

Commission E suggests the following standard mixture as a **"stomach tea"** for loss of appetite, dyspeptic symptoms such as sensation of fullness and flatulence, mild spastic symptoms in the gastrointestinal region:

Rp	Angelicae radix conc.	20.0 g
	Gentianae radix conc.	40.0 g
	Carvi fructus tot.	40.0 g

M. f. species stomachicae
Dosage: Up to 3 cups daily before meals, made using a heaped teaspoonful of the mixture. Some children will complain of the bitter taste, but the mixture is highly effective.

3.3.3 Indigestion

It is evident from Tables 1 and 2 that basically almost 40 plant drugs are suitable for treating indigestion in the widest sense. Below, only the **mild forms of indigestion** seen in infants and children will be considered. **A warning:** Transition to severe types with **toxicosis** tends to be gradual; caution is indicated especially if the symptoms go hand in hand with pyrexia. Minor forms of indigestion are usually acute nutritional disorders caused by moderate enteric infections. Potential pathogens include viruses, above all rotaviruses, staphylococci, Pyocyaneus, Proteus, Shigella, Salmonella, Campylobacter, pathogens of the TPE group, Yersinia and, relatively uncommon, "dyspepsia colibacteria".

The **symptoms** are:

- Loss of appetite and even refusing food
- general restlessness
- failure to gain weight
- flatulence
- meteorism
- diarrhoea ("fermentative stools")
- vomiting

The treatments available for loss of appetite were discussed in the previous section.

3.3.4 Flatulence and Meteorism

A number of effective carminative vegetable drugs are available for the treatment of **flatulence** (= passing increased amounts of intestinal gases via the anus) and **meteorism** (= excessive amounts of gases in the gastrointestinal tract which may cause distension). The volatile oil drugs of the Apioideae subfamily of the Umbelliferae, anise, fennel and caraway merit first consideration.

Anise fruit, **Anisi fructus** (botanical name *Pimpinella anisum* L.), **fennel fruit**, **Foeniculi fructus** (botanical name *Foeniculum vulgare* Miller) and **caraway fruit**, **Carvi fructus** (botanical name *Carum carvi* L.). Equal parts of these three are used for the **"AFC tea"** that is proving of great value in dealing with flatulence in Medical Unit B at Rissen-Hamburg Hospital. Another equally well tried and tested method is to rub pure **caraway oil** or a 10% solution of Carvi aetheroleum in olive oil into the abdomen, especially the umbilical region.

The following **"caraway drops"** have also proved effective:

Rp Carvi aetheroleum 2.0
   Valerianae aeth. tinct. 10.0
   Tinct. carminativa 10.0
M.D.S. three times daily 10−20 drops after meals in herb tea or fruit juice. Not for children less than 1 year old.

The various **"wind ointments"** should not be forgotten for the treatment of infants. Apart from the volatile oils of the above Umbelliferae fruits they also contain basil oil (*Ocimum basilicum* L.), cherry laurel oil (*Prunus laurocerasus* L.) or marjoram oil (*Origanum majorana* L.), especially as Unguentum Majorani. Quick and easy to use is the Tinctura carminativa in the Supplement to the *Ger. P.* 6. The formula for the proprietary Carminativum Hetterich® is based on the pharmacopoeial formula and has proved its value. [68]

Finally reference should be made to the following suggestion for a **"wind tea"** based on the Commission E guidelines for standard combinations:

Matricariae flos conc.	30.0 g
Menthae piperitae folium conc.	15.0 g
Carvi fructus cont.	20.0 g
Foeniculi fructus cont.	30.0 g
Aurantii pericarpium conc.	5.0 g

Dosage: Depending on severity, several times daily a cupful of the wind tea, made with 2 teaspoonfuls of Species deflatulentes, as an infusion. For infants, 50−100 ml given in the feeding bottle are recommended.

The tea mixture has a pleasant taste and is accepted even by infants.

It is important to know, however, that

- anise may occasionally cause allergic reactions (sensitivity to anethol) and
- mothers must be told that Umbelliferae fruits need to be crushed (using a spoon) immediately before the infusion is made. The reason is that the active principles are contained in deep excretory ducts in these fruits.

For schoolchildren, the Commission E standard "stomach tea" mixture (p. 48) would also be suitable.

3.3.5 Diarrhoea

Commission E has so far approved 7 monographs of plant drugs suitable for the treatment of short-term diarrhoea (Table 3). The following note has been included to good purpose in the monographs: "A doctor must be consulted if the diarrhoea persists for more than 3 or 4 days."

Substitution of water and electrolytes is clearly the most important step, followed by dietary measures. In cases of acute diarrhoea and vomiting, no solid food is given but a 5% glucose solution (as glucose tea or one of the commercially available glucose and electrolyte solu-

Table 3. Phytotherapeutic drugs indicated for diarrhoea (Commission E)

● Agrimoniae herba ● Alchemillae herba ● Coffeae carbo ● Myrtilli fructus ● Quercus cortex ● Syzygii cumini cortex ● Tormentillae rhizoma
These drugs are only suitable for **nonspecific acute diarrhoea** (mainly the type known as "summer" diarrhoea) **Caution:** If diarrhoea persists for more than 3 or 4 days, a doctor must be consulted. This applies particularly if the patient also has a temperature. Basic treatment always consists in water and electrolyte substitution.

Presentations ● Powdered medicinal herb (!), particularly effective
             ● Aqueous extracts
             ● Ethanolic tinctures (not for infants)
             ● Dry extracts

tions), soon supplementing this with a pectin preparation such as Aplona®, Apfeldiät Granulat (apple diet granulate) or Diarrhoesan®.

Infants and young children should never be given **loperamide** (e.g. Imodium®) unless it has been prescribed for them. The drug is certainly suitable for adults to take as self-medication for acute or traveller's diarrhoea, [92] but it is a powerful motility inhibitor and should only be given to children under strict medical supervision, ideally by a paediatrician.[93] American physicians have developed a detailed posology especially for children.

The most suitable plant antidiarrhoeics are dried **bilberries, Myrtilli fructus** (botanical name *Vaccinium myrtillus* L.). A relatively high-dose aqueous extract has to be made of these. Parents frequently tend to disregard this and then report failure. The mean daily dose must be 30 g of the dried berries.

Pour about 400 ml of hot water on 3 heaped tablespoonfuls of Myrtilli fructus and simmer on a low flame for about 10 minutes. Providing the daily dose of 30 g of the dried berries is not exceeded, there can be no overdosage at any age group. Patients are given the above extract made from 30 g of the dried berries to drink ad libitum throughout the day.

The second plant drug to be considered is **coffee charcoal, Coffeae carbo** (botanical names *Coffea arabica* L., *Coffea liberica* Bull ex Hiern, *Coffea canephora* Pierre ex Froehner). Compared to bilberries it has adsorptive capacity and is therefore liable to interfere with the absorption of other drugs given simultaneously. According to the Commission E Monograph, the mean daily dose to treat nonspecific acute diarrhoea is about 9 g.

The "diarrhoea remedy" every mother has immediately at hand is **tea, Theae folium** (botanical name *Camellia* *sinensis* Kuntze, O.). It is not widely known, however, that unfermented green tea is much more effective than the fermented black tea. Unfortunately green tea is not always to the children's taste. They will generally accept the semi-fermented oolong tea, which is also superior to black tea for antidiarrhoeic action. As a "diarrhoea remedy" the tea has to be left to infuse for about 15 minutes, using a heaped teaspoonful per cup.

A number of earlier clinical papers [80] from paediatric hospitals and practices and a more recent study from a children"s hospital [81] report good results with both diarrhoea and diarrhoea and vomiting in children from the use of Liquor Uzara or a standardized "Uzara" dry extract (see p. 53 for proprietary products). **Liquor Uzara** is an ethanolic extract of the root of *Xysmalobium undulatum* (L.) R. Brown, a plant native to South Africa. Commission E gives nonspecific, acute diarrhoeas under Indications for **Uzara root (Uzarae radix)**.

The drug contains glycosides with cardenolide structure (e.g. uzarigenin), so that it is essential to use a standardized proprietary product in paediatrics (see p. 53). The exact posology for children is stated on the package. Several authors [80] report no undesirable side effects in children even with adult doses. This should not tempt us to go beyond the doses recommended for children.

Excellent clinical results have also been seen with Saccharomyces Boulardii preparations. The antagonistic effect on undesirable microorganisms, neutralization of bacterial toxins and influence on the association immune system are completely different principles of action. Efficacy has been demonstrated in a double-blind trial with 130 children [102].

3.3.6 Habitual constipation

Chronic constipation is more common among children and young people than is generally assumed.

Possible causes include:

- faulty diet
- wrong eating habits
- adiposity (may be "pre-programmed" from infancy)
- suppression of defecation reflex, e.g. at nursery school or school and when travelling
- fear of pain if anal rhagades, fissures, haemorrhoids are present
- psychosomatic factors, e.g. fear of getting fat (especially in girls), school stress, examination nerves.

For treatment, the first step is to consider removing the causes. For medical treatment, physicians and pharmacists should give more thought to the alternatives to the anthranoid laxatives. Table 4 gives a brief overview of the alternatives.

The first drug to be considered is **linseed, Lini semen** (botanical name *Linum usitatissimum* L.). The Commission E Monograph lists habitual constipation, colon impaired by laxative abuse, irritable colon, diverticulitis; mucilage for gastritis and enteritis under indications. Failures or inadequate results are generally due to wrong use and/or linseed of poor pharmaceutical quality.

For treatment to be successful, the linseed used must have a swelling index of not less than 5. The swelling index of 4 given in the *Ger. P.* 10 is usually too low. It is not for nothing that paediatricians report good results with the proprietary products Linusit®-Creola or Linusit®-Gold but find linseed as such unsatisfactory. The linseed used for

Table 4. Alternatives to anthranoid-containing laxatives

1) Laxatives with osmotic action
a) salinic laxatives (e.g. Karlsbad salt)   b) carbohydrates that are not easily absorbed (e.g. mannitol)
2) Laxatives that act via the dilatation stimulus = bulking agents

a) Lini semen
   b) Psyllii semen
   c) tragacanth, pectins, carmellose, etc.
   d) "ballast" (e.g. bran, fruit fibre)

3) Laxatives with microbiological activity

a) lactose
   b) lactose + milk protein in combination
   c) lactulose
   d) intestinal bacteria

Linusit® preparations has been specially grown and has a swelling index of 6−10. The second important aspect is that adequate amounts of fluids must be taken at the same time. The ground rule is a proportion of 1:10, i.e. take about 150 ml of fluid to every tablespoonful of linseed. This will achieve the increase in volume needed to effect the dilatation stimulus in the intestinal wall. The third point to be noted is that coarse ground linseed may swell up too early, i.e. in the stomach. A clinical trial [82] has shown that whole or lightly cracked (Linusit® method) linseed is more effective than coarse ground. It has also shown that it is more effective to take linseed between rather than during meals.

Flea or plantago seed, Psyllii semen (botanical name *Plantago psyllium* L.) is also listed for "habitual chronic constipation and irritable colon" by Commission E. Allergic reactions have been reported – though only on rare occasions –, powdered flea seed tends to adhere unpleasantly between the teeth, and may increase flatulence and distension when first used, so that flea seed is not likely to be much used in paediatrics. Some paediatricians have, however, reported good results with the proprietary Agiocur®, a flea seed preparation based on a granulate. A number of other proprietary products containing flea seed (see p. 53) also do not have the undesirable properties of pure flea seed.

A useful and highly recommended measure is to give children high-fibre fruit or bran bars to take to school rather than biscuits or sandwiches.

If the use of **anthranoid laxatives** is inevitable, the drug of first choice in paediatrics would be frangula bark, **Frangulae cortex** (botanical name *Rhamnus frangula* L.) and Chinese rhubarb, **Rhei radix** (botanical names *Rheum palmatum* L . and *Rheum officinale* Baillon). It is important **not** to fall back on **aloes, Aloe**, or **senna leaves or fruit, Senna folium or fructus**. Mono-

Table 5. Toxicology/side effects of laxatives with "chemical action" – Review
(anthranoids, bisacodyl, sodium picosulphate, phenolphthalein, etc.)

1) So far (1994) nothing further is known about the vicious circle of
   a) habituation
   b) loss of electrolytes (above all potassium)
   that might possibly exonerate these drugs.

2) Recent discoveries relating to anthranoids:
   a) Melanosis coli = reversible, clinically not relevant
   b) Danthron side effects do not apply to anthranoids as regards
      • damage to neuromuscular apparatus of colon
      • genotoxic effects
      • carcinogenic or co-carcinogenic effects
   c) Anthranoids in mother's milk?
      Exonerating studies are not convincing; therefore contraindicated whilst breast-feeding
   d) Anthranoid extracts have a lower LD_{50} than pure anthranoids, i.e. pure sennosides are better tolerated.

graphs for all five drugs are available. Anthranoid laxatives differ not only in their actions but also in their side effects (see Tables 5 and 6), and pharmacists should not only be well informed but also have reasonable knowledge concerning the composition of the proprietary products. Table 7 offers some guidance.

3.3.7 Proprietary Products

a) **Loss of appetite**
Anorex® Appetit Tropfen, Blüten (flower) Pollen Fink, pollisynergen capsules
b) **Gastrointestinal spasms and inflammation**
Kamillosan® Lösung, Kamille® Spitzner, Perkamillon® Liquidum, Salus® Kamillentropfen, Salus®, Salus® Kamillentee tea bags
c) **Flatulence and meteorism**
Unguentum Majorani, Unguentum Aromaticum *Austr. P.*, Babyluuf Balsam, Pekana Blähungssalbe (flatulence ointment), Windsalbe Taminy-line, Mentacur® capsules (if school age)

d) **Diarrhoea**
Aplona® Granulat, Uzara® coated tablets and solution, entero sanol® juice, Oralpädon® tablets, Perenterol® capsules
e) **Acute constipation**
(containing anthranoids)
Liquidepur® liquid, Bekunis® chocolate, Neda® fruit cubes, Pursennid® coated tablets
f) **Chronic constipation**
Linusit® Creola, Linusit® Gold, Agiocur® granulate, Bio Bekunis® granulate, Psyllium Kneipp powder, Metamucil® powder, Puraya® granulate

Table 6. Possible classifications of anthranoid drugs – Review

1) According to laxative effect • aloes • senna leaves • senna fruit, cascara bark • frangula bark • rhubarb root	most powerful effect ↓ weakest effect
2) According to undesirable side effects in form of abdominal colics • aloes • senna leaves • cascara bark • senna fruit • frangula bark • rhubarb root • pure senna glycosides and • purified senna extracts	most powerful side effect ↓ weakest side effect

3) According to major contraindications
 aloes   • in pregnancy
        • during menstrual periods
        • with inflammatory pelvic
          conditions
	Reason: Abdominal vessels in whole pelvic region well filled with blood

4) According to chemical composition a) Anthrone drugs, e.g. aloes > senna leaves and fruit > cascara bark b) Anthraquinone drugs, e.g. frangula bark > rhubarb root c) Anthranoid glycosides: relative to concentration of free anthrones and/or anthraquinones	

Table 7. Possible pharmaceutical classification of anthranoid laxatives – Review

1) Monopreparations e.g. aloes (e.g. Jacobus Schwedenkräutermischung [Swedish herb mixture]) senna leaves and fruit (e.g. Bekunis® preparations) senna fruit extracts (e.g. Depuran®) pure sennosides (e.g. Pursenid®)
2) Compound preparations a) with aloes (e.g. M-40 coated tablets, Daluwal, Dragees 19 [coated tablets], etc.) b) without aloes (e.g. Tirgon coated tablets, Wörishofner Abführtabletten [laxative tablets]) c) without aloes and with bulking agents (e.g. Agiolax®, Normacol®) d) anthranoids plus bisacodyl (e.g. Daluwal forte, Tirgon coated tablets)
3) Standardized or not standardized? a) Total anthranoid content stated b) Individual anthranoids listed (e.g. sennoside), required by Commission E (1994)

3.4 Urogenital Disorders

3.4.1 Urinary Tract Infections

Infections of the kidney and lower urinary tract are among the most common bacterial infections in childhood. [70, 71] Among the newborn, boys are 2 or 3 times as frequently affected than girls, but later on girls have the condition up to 20 times more frequently. The genesis of urinary tract infection is not clearly established, which is one main reason why people should be advised against self-medication unless a definite diagnosis has been made. Above all it is necessary to establish if the infection involves the lower urinary tract only or the upper tract as well (pyelonephritis). Anatomical abnormalities that might impede flow must also be excluded.

Once the infection has been diagnosed by establishing the organisms in a midstream or catheter urine specimen and testing for resistance (Escherichia coli, Proteus, Klebsiella and Pseudomonas are the most commonly found pathogens) immediate chemotherapy is usually required (e.g. trimethoprim/sulphamethoxazole, ampillicin, cephalosporins, gyrase inhibitors).

Phytotherapy also has a great deal to offer for urinary tract inflammation:

1 Measures to prevent reinfection and recurrences, such as irrigation therapy, are the first to be considered.
2) In second place comes the treatment of isolated covert bacteriuria. This does not involve leukocyturia or pyrexia, pain in the side, etc. Antibiotics may be held in reserve to begin with, [70] providing there are no appreciable symptoms (temperature, disinclination to take fluids, vomiting, severe pain at urination) nor microbial data to indicate a need for antibiotics (e.g. bacterial count in midstream urine > 10^5/ml).

In either case irrigation is indicated with extracts of single or mixtures of herbal drugs that ideally have the following actions:

disinfectant
antiinflammatory and antipyretic
aquaretic.

Individual plant drugs do not fully cover the necessary spectrum of action, so that urologists tend to use combinations in form of teas or standard multi-ingredient preparations. Reputable urologists hold the view that irrigation with a kidney or bladder tea is not merely a rational method of treatment but also saves costs.

Disinfectant plant drugs include **bearberry leaves, cowberry (red whortleberry) leaves, bergenia leaves, sweet sumach bark and watercress or nasturtium (capuchin cress) herb**. A steam distillate of nasturtium has the greatest antibacterial activity. The resulting benzyl mustard oil, a liquid with a strong odour of cress, has been shown to be effective against gram-positive and -negative organisms. A proprietary preparation of it (see p. 58) has proved its value particularly with candida infections of the lower urinary tract. Care must be taken with children that they do not bite into the soft capsules but swallow them whole after meals.

A herbal preparation that is widely used, also for self-medication, and has been shown to have disinfectant properties is **bearberry leaves, Uvae ursi folium** (botanical name *Arctostaphylos uva ursi* L.). Aqueous extracts are rather tart and therefore not popular with children if given on their own. They may however be used in combination with other plant drugs.

The Commission E Monograph gives the following indications for Uvae ursi folium: "Inflammatory conditions of lower urinary tract". The recommended daily dose for adequate disinfectant effect is about 10 g of the leaves or preparations containing 400–700 mg of arbutin. Multi-ingredient preparations do not reach that level, yet clinical trials have shown some of them to be efficacious. [57]

Bearberry leaf preparations only have disinfectant action if the urine is slightly alkaline. This presents another problem in paediatrics. In adults the necessary alkalinity is achieved by giving sodium bicarbonate (baking soda). In paediatrics, a high fluid intake is required to make up for any deficiency (2–3 litres a day); this will naturally reduce the number of organisms. To put it plainly, it means that kidney and bladder teas used in paediatrics must **taste good**.

This criterion is met not only by sugar-agglomerate teas (e.g. TAD Harntee (urinary tea) 400 or Dr Klinger's Bergischer Kräutertee (herb tea), for a clinical trial has shown that tea bags are also effective (e.g. Uro Fink® Tea). The question is, of course, if our efforts should go so far that the products consist to 96% of refined sugar and only 4% of medicinal plant extracts. When it comes to pharmaceutical evaluation, the issue is obviously clear.

Reference should be made at this point to the warning issued by the German Federal Government's in 1985 that children's teas containing sugar and carbohydrate cause caries.[59] The public were informed that sugared teas, irrespective of whether they were sold as medicines or food, could cause, or at least support the development of caries if given to infants and young children for any length of time.

Kidney and bladder teas for children

Betulae folium conc.	20.0 g
Orthosiphonis folium conc.	20.0 g
Solidaginis herba conc.	25.0 g
Uvae ursi folium conc.	30.0 g
Menthae piperitae folium conc.	5.0 g

Dosage: 1 cupful up to 5 times a day, made with a heaped teaspoonful to 1 tablespoonful of the mixture, leaving to infuse for 10 minutes.

Combination **without** bearberry leaves:

Orthosiphonis folium conc.	30.0 g
Ononidis radix conc.	15.0 g
Solidaginis herba conc.	20.0 g
Rhois aromaticae cortex conc.	30.0 g
Aurantii pericarpium conc.	5.0 g

Dosage: 1 cupful up to 3 times daily, using a tablespoonful of the mixture as an infusion.

3.4.2 Enuresis nocturna and diurna

The second major area for phytotherapy in **diseases of the bladder** in childhood is the adjuvant treatment of **enuresis nocturna and diurna**. Bedwetting and the inability to be continent in the daytime are up to 50% psychological. The first step must therefore be to create a new, sounder basis by naturopathic methods. [5] Pharmacists should draw attention to this before dispensing medicaments for the condition. Other useful measures would be to reduce fluid intake in the afternoon and evening, avoidance of spices that cause kidney irritation, and an early supper.

Phytotherapy might help to strengthen the sphincter and provide mild sedation, e.g. with Hyperforat® drops. [79] **Pumpkin seed, Cucurbitae peponis**

Table 8. Rationale for combination?

Indication
• Irritable bladder due to functional and/or organic causes (1st and 2nd degree) • Enuresis nocturna and/or diurna

Constituents

1) Extr. Cort. Rhois aromaticae radicis	(sweet sumach root bark)
2) Extr. Fol. Uvae ursi (stand. for not less than 20% of arbutin)	(bearberry leaves)
3) Lipophilic extract of Cucurbitae semen c.v. peponis medicinalis	("medicinal" pumpkin seed)
4) Extr. Rad. Piperis Methystici (stand. for not less than 25% Kawain)	(kava kava root)
5) Extr. Flor. Lupuli	(hop strobiles)

Clinical trials
• urgency reduced
• incontinence improved
• excessive diurnal and nocturnal frequency reduced
• dysuria relieved or improved

Actions of drug extracts 1−5

1) antiinflammatory and bacteriostatic	popular medicine only
2) disinfectant	
3) improving muscle tone in bladder	experimental and/or clinical
4) anticonvulsant	proof (monographs)
5) sedative	

semen (botanical name *Cucurbita pepo* L.) is the only Monograph with the indications "**Irritable bladder**, dysuria with benign prostatic hyperplasia" to have been passed by Commission E. Only the seeds of *Cucurbita pepo* L. convar. *citrullinina* Greb. var. *styriaca* Greb. have been tested, however.

3.4.3 Irritable Bladder

In the treatment of **irritable bladder** and also enuresis nocturna, good results have been achieved with the proprietary product Granufink® Kürbis (pumpkin) Granulat.[60] This consists of the granulated and sugar-coated seed of a pumpkin specially grown for medicinal pur-

poses.[61] Children like to take it and it is easy to add to foods (e.g. yoghurt, muesli, fruit salads, puddings, etc.), so that there are no problems with compliance.

Positive clinical results have also been reported with Cysto-Fink® capsules.[62] These are a size suitable for children and were taken without problems.

Table 8 gives an overview of clinical findings and also presents an attempt to make the standard combination plausible, in line with the Commission E guidelines. The available multi-ingredient preparation should meet drugs legislation requirements and therefore continue to be available as a tried and tested preparation for paediatric use.

3.4.4 Proprietary Products

a) **Irrigation therapy**
Blasen- und Nierentee (bladder & kidney tea) Stada®, Buccosperin Tea, Folindor Tea, Uro-Fink® tea bags
Uroflux® powdered bladder and kidney tea, Solubitrat® powdered bladder and kidney tea, Nierentee (kidney tea) 2000 powder, Niron Tee powder

b) **Infection/inflammation mainly of lower urinary tract in form of isolated covert bacteriuria**
Angocin coated tablets, Arctuvan® cotated tablets, Canephron® drops, Cefanephrin® N drops, Cystinol solution, Cystinol mono coated tablets, Gelosantol® capsules, Tromacaps® Capsules (no longer available since 1992 for purely pharmaceutical reasons), Uraton drops, Uvalysat® Bürger drops

c) **Irritable bladder and enuresis**
Cysto-Fink® capsules, Cystinol solution, Enuresibletten coated tablets, Granufink® granulate, Hicoton tablets, Hyperforat® drops, Urgenin® Liquidum

3.5 Psychosomatic Disorders

Phytotherapeutic treatment of conditions that are psychological in origin ranks high in paediatrics. On one hand the incidence is steadily increasing and on the other psychotropic synthetic drugs, especially the benzodiazepines, must be used as little as possible in paediatrics. The ideal is, of course, to avoid tranquillizers of the benzodiazepine type altogether, and phytotherapy has much to offer in this respect.

Common complaints are

- General nervousness and restlessness
- Lack of concentration
- Anxiety states
- Problems going to sleep and sleeping through the night
- Nervous palpitations
- Nervous excitation
- Nervous stomach pain coupled with loss of appetite

Before considering specific phytotherapeutic measures it should be stressed that medication of any kind, irrespective of whether it consists of synthetic sedatives and psychotropic drugs or phytomedicines, should always only be the second step. Careful analysis of problems and causes as the basis for a warm, human approach to the child or young person should be the first step in treating the condition.[96] Medicaments, of any form whatever, cannot replace genuine concern and the effort to solve the problem and deal with the causes; it is, of course, not uncommon for the effort not to be made.[96, 101]

3.5.1 Sedatives
(Restlessness, Anxiety States, Sleep Disorders)

The plant world provides a considerable range of psychotropic drugs with anxiolytic, antidepressant, antipsychotic and also thymoleptic activities, though the intensity and time pattern of actions do not compare with those of synthetic psychotropic drugs. This "gap in herbal medicine", as Prof. Weiss calls it in chapter 11 of his textbook, [1] might be said to be predestined for paediatrics.

Valerian root, Valerianae radix (botanical name *Valeriana officinalis* (several forms) L.) is held in high regard in phytotherapy for its sedative properties, but in paediatrics valerian tea or tincture play only a minor role. The reason is that children generally refuse it on account of the odour and taste. They will, however, accept valerian preparations (proprietary products, see p. 62) in form of coated tablets or soft gelatin capsules.

The Commission E Monograph for valerian root lists "restless states, problems going to sleep due to nervous causes" under Indications. It explicitly states that these indications are for preparations **not containing valepotriates**.

Potential side effects of valepotriates are currently under discussion.[63] Valepotriates have epoxide structure and are therefore alkylating agents, their alkylating potential comparable to that of epichlorohydrin, a powerful chemical mutagen and carcinogen.[64] For safety's sake, only valepotriate- and baldrinal-free valerian preparations should be used in paediatrics. Baldrinals are dienetype degradation products of valepotriates. They are not found in the plant itself. In the SOS chromotest they, too, show genotoxicity and bactericidal properties.[65]

Recent investigations by Dieckmann [65] have shown that a number of proprietary products (see p. 62) contain **neither valepotriates nor baldrinals**. This would certainly be the case if those products were made with aqueous dry extracts of *Valeriana officinalis* roots. With the usual method of making valerian tea, practically no valepotriate is extracted from the plant drug. Added to this is the fact that the valepotriate concentration in officinal European valerian root is quite low at 0.006−0,9%.

The most important outcome of Dieckmann's dissertation [65] is the discovery that the **mutagenic properties of valepotriates and baldrinals are lost** almost immediately, as these compounds are rapidly metabolized in the body. The metabolites Dieckmann isolated were baldrinal glucuronides which did not give positive results in the Ames or the SOS chromotest. These are extremely important findings that will to some extent allay anxieties in assessing potential risks. They should not be taken as a general "all-clear", however. In theory, there is a residual risk for the gastrointestinal tract until the compounds are metabolized, even if it has not been possible to demonstrate free valepotriates or baldrinals in the blood or other organs. Long-term *in vivo* studies will be needed to clarify the situation.

Critical assessment of all the facts may lead to the conclusion that for **adults**, medicines containing valepotriates offer greater benefit than risk compared to the abuse of synthetic psychotropic drugs. [104]

In **paediatrics**, however, it is important to give only valepotriate- and baldrinal-free valerian preparations. One of these is valerian tea (pour 200 ml of boiling water over 1 teaspoonful of minced valerian root and leave to infuse for 15 minutes). Valerian tincture, Valerianae tinctura *Ger. P.* 10 may also be safely used (from 3 years onwards, 1/2 teaspoonful in milk or fruit juice before bedtime).

For reasons of taste and odour, cold macerations (extract Valerianae radix conc. for at least 8 hours in cold water, at room temperature) would also be suitable. In popular medicine they are actually considered to be more efficacious.

Systematic investigations to substantiate this are still outstanding.

Standardized valerian preparations that have been through clinical trials are of course specially recommended (proprietary products, p. 62). Clinical trials of Valdispert® coated tablets have been made not only with adults but also specifically with children.[84−88] Apart from confirming the above indications in the Commission E Monograph, they also provided additional indications. F. Wurst [87] has reported interesting results in schoolchildren with anxiety-based learning difficulties.

Valerianae radix is most commonly combined with

- hop cones (strobiles), Lupuli strobulus (botanical name *Humulus lupulus* L.)
- balm leaves, Melissae folium (botanical name *Melissa officinalis* L.)
- lavender flowers, Lavandulae flos (botanical name *Lavandula angustifolia* Miller)
- passion flower herb, Passiflorae herba (botanical name *Passiflora incarnata* L.).

Monographs on all the four above are available and also cover the posology (see appendix).

The indications given for **hops** are: "Psychosomatic conditions such as restlessness and anxiety states, sleep disorders". For 1 cup of hop tea, pour 1/4 litre of boiling water on to 1 tablespoonful of hop strobiles and leave to infuse for 10 minutes. Up to the age of three, 1 cup per day is usually sufficient, after this the dose may be increased to 1 cup 3 times daily.

The indications for **balm leaves** are: "Problems going to sleep of nervous origin, functional gastrointestinal disorders".

For 1 cup of balm tea, pour about 150 ml of boiling water on to 1 tablespoonful of cut-up balm leaves, cover the container and leave to infuse for about 10 minutes. Infants are given 1 cup in divided doses over the day, young children up to 3 cups daily.

The indications given for **lavender flowers** are: "Psychosomatic conditions such as restlessness, problems going to sleep, functional epigastric symptoms, nervous stomach and intestinal symptoms due to nerves". Dosage: Pour 150 ml of boiling water on to 1 teaspoonful of lavender flowers, cover, and leave to infuse for 10 minutes.

The use given for **passion flower herb** is: "nervous restlessness".

Dosage: Pour 150−200 ml of boiling water on to 1 tablespoonful of the cut-up herb and infuse on a low flame for 5 minutes. Young children are given 1 cup per day, children of 3 years and over, up to 3 cups daily.

The **sedative properties** of the four plant drugs have been fully substantiated [104] including their use in paediatrics. There are, however, organoleptic reasons why the emphasis varies. There are also different or additional methods of use.

A tea made entirely of **hop strobiles** is not exactly popular with children, especially if made with "pharmaceutical" hops that have been stored. These smell of isovaleric acid and differ markedly from fresh "beer hops" in their 2-methyl-3-butene-2-ol concentration. "Beer hops" have an aromatic, slightly balsamic odour. 2-Methyl-3-buten-2-ol is a C_5 alcohol produced due to autoxidation of the bitter principles on storage. The methylbutenol is a volatile compound and probably responsible for the therapeutic action of **"hop pillows"**, a tried and tested household remedy for

restless infants and **young children**. They are made by filling a cotton or linen bag with about 500 g of hop strobiles and using this as a pillow. The filling may be used for about a week.

It has been shown in animal trials that methylbutenol has marked sedative and hypnotic activity [66] and that this is dose-dependent. Comparison of hops with Allotropal® (3-methyl-1-pentin-3-ol) confirmed the usefulness of pharmaceutical hops as aromatherapy.

A similar type of aromatherapy is applied in the South of France where **bunches or bags of lavender flowers** are hung up near the child's cot. **Lavender baths** have also proved of value (proprietary products, p. 62). They may be prepared by using an infusion of Lavandulae flos or adding a proprietary lavender preparation. Pour 1−2 litres of boiling water on to 50−100 g of lavender flowers and leave to infuse for 10 minutes. Use the whole quantity to one full bath, which should take 15 minutes. Recent investigations [106] have confirmed the sedative and hypnotic properties of volatile oil of lavender.

Balm leaves are used either in **balm tea**, which children like to take, or as aqueous, ethanolic or oily extracts in baths. Oily extracts offer the highest quality. The various cordials (Melissengeist) on the market are not suitable for internal use in paediatrics because of their high alcohol content (usually > 70% v/v). On the other hand it is perfectly alright to add 5−15 drops of Melissengeist to a full bath for balneotherapy.

A **herbal sedative** that has attracted attention thanks to recent clinical and experimental studies is **St. John's wort, Hyperici herba** (botanical name *Hypericum perforatum* L.). Controlled and double blind trials have shown it to have effects comparable to those of diazepam in adults. The conclusion drawn from this is that St John's wort preparations may be a reliable alternative to the commonly used synthetic drugs in treating mild to medium severe depression. The trials also showed improvement in nervous restlessness and sleep disorders. The excellent antibacterial and antiinflammatory activities of St John's wort have already been discussed (p. 25ff). Biflavonoids of the apigenin type, and especially amentoflavones and xanthones, may be responsible for the sedative effect, as these natural compounds show a remarkable degree of binding to the diazepam receptor. There are many reasons why it seems reasonable to use *Hypericum perforatum* also in paediatrics. [89]

To make St. John's wort tea, put about 200 ml of boiling water on to 1 teaspoonful of the cut-up herb (the proportion of stems should be as low as possible) and leave to infuse for 10 minutes. Young children are given 1 cupful, children above 3 years of age may be given 2 or 3 cups per day. Hypericins cause photosensitization but aqueous extracts contain only small amounts of these. It is, however, advisable to avoid direct exposure to the sun immediately after taking the tea.

St. John's wort fluidextract (Extractum Hyperici fluidum) is also recommended. Recommended dose: young children 5 drops 2 x daily, schoolchildren 10 drops up to 3 times daily. Standardized proprietary products may be used (see p. 62) to treat depressive states in young people.

Sedative tea for children
(Species nervinae pro infantibus)

Melissae folium conc.	30.0 g
Lavandulae flos tot.	30.0 g

Passiflorae herba conc.	30.0 g
Hyperici herba conc.	10.0 g

Dosage: According to age, 1−3 cups daily. For 1 cup, pour about 200 ml of boiling water on to 1 tablespoonful of the mixture.

Sedative tea – standard Commission E mixture

Valerianae radix conc.	40.0 g
Passiflorae herba conc.	30.0 g
Melissae folium conc.	30.0 g

Dosage: Up to 5 cups daily, made with a heaped teaspoonful of the mixture.

Finally attention should be drawn to a medicinal plant of which Commission E has published a negative report as regards the constituents (due to the absence of well-documented clinical reports). It is nevertheless widely used as a sedative for children by paediatricians, especially those versed in homoeopathy. **Eschscholtzia californica** Chamisso, the Californian poppy, is much more widely known as a children's sedative in North America than in Europe. The homoeopathic mother tincture, in pharmaceutical terms really a conventional pharmaceutical preparation, is most commonly used, as is the proprietary product Phytonoxon N tincture (the German Homoeopathic Pharmacopoeia Commission has not yet produced a monograph on *Eschscholtzia*). Recent pharmacological trials of aqueous extracts from the aerial parts of *Eschscholtzia californica* showed significant sedative and anxiolytic effects in mice.[94] Californian poppy, a traditional medicinal herb in North America, has therefore also gained the interest of pharmacologists.

Standardized preparations of Kava-kava (from the rhizome of *Piper methysticum* Forster) have recently been shown to have useful anxiolytic properties and may also be of interest in paediatrics. A Commission E Monograph is available.

3.5.2 Proprietary Products

a) **Valepotriate-free valerian monopreparations**
Baldrian Phyton® coated tablets, Florabio Baldrian-Frischpflanzenpreßsaft, Kneipp® Baldrian-Pflanzensaft, Recvalysat® Bürger drops, Sedalint-Baldrian (valerian) tablets, Valdispert® coated tablets

b) **Valepotriate-free valerian multiingredient preparations**
Euvegal® coated tablets N, Hova® Kinder (paediatric) suppositories, Hovaletten coated tablets, Ivel-Sleeping coated tablets, Luvased coated tablets, Moradorm S filmcoated tablets, Münchner Baldrian Perlen, Plantival® drops, Valdispert® comp. coated tablets

c) **Lavender preparations**
Kneipp® Lavender bath, Kneipp® Lavender bath salts, Salus Nervenbad, Weleda® Lavender Bath Lotion

d) **St. John's Wort mono- and multiingredient preparations**
Hyperforat® drops, Jarsin® coated tablets, Kneipp® Johanniskraut (St. John's wort) Pflanzensaft, Neuroplant capsules, Psychotonin® M drops, Psychatrin® Jossa coated tablets, Sedariston® drops and capsules.

3.6 Analgesia

Analgesics are given rather indiscriminately to children and young people, which lays the foundations for drug abuse and analgesics dependency. Herbal analgesics do not compare with "classic" analgesics such as acetylsalicylic acid, paracetamol, mefenamic acid, flufenamic acid, metamizole, propyphenazone and ibuprofen; nor are they able to block the pain centre in the brain.

Phytotherapy nevertheless offers a number of natural substances or preparations that can ameliorate or remove the following types of pain:

- tension headache (myogelosis)
- acute toothache or wound pain
- pain in extremities with colds and influenza
- psychogenic headaches
- attacks of migraine.

3.6.1 Tension Headaches

Tension or vasomotor headaches generally involve dysregulation of vascular tone in the head region. The first steps in treatment should be relaxation exercises and massage to loosen the muscles in the neck and shoulder region. Some relief may also be gained from blocking excitation of peripheral pain receptors by a kind of "superficial or infiltration anaesthesia". This is sometimes successfully done by applying a few drops of peppermint or mint oil. Proprietary products (see p. 64) have proved effective in treating purely **functional** vasoconstriction.

3.6.2 Wound Pain

The **pain of injuries, especially blunt trauma** (contusions, bruises, etc.), is also relieved by applying a *few* drops of peppermint or mint oil. If menthol sprays are used, care must be taken to see that the menthol content is not more than 5%. If it is too high, peripheral pain receptors may be sensitized so that pain on pressure increases.

For this reason, it would be better not to use pure peppermint or mint oil, as in the clinical trials,[32, 36] but a 10% oily solution. Miglyol® or Freiöl® are particularly suitable diluents.

3.6.3 Toothache

For **acute toothache**, e.g. due to caries, a plug of cotton wool or cotton thread soaked in oil of cloves (Caryophylli aetheroleum *Ger. P.* 10) is a tried and tested family remedy. Such a measure must always be short-term, of course, and a visit to the dentist should follow as soon as possible. Caryophylli aetheroleum has both local anaesthetic and disinfectant properties.

This "family medicine" has now also gone through clinical trials, which confirm the results known from popular medicine (see Monograph in Appendix).

3.6.4 Pain in Extremities

Pain in the extremities during colds and influenza responds to **willow bark**, aspen leaves or meadowsweet flowers or standardized proprietary products made from them (see p. 63). For details see the section on Colds (p. 41). The medicinal action – known from empirical medicine and to some extent substantiated in clinical and experimental studies – is clearly due to inhibition of prostaglandin synthesis by salicin derivatives. In a way this presents sensitization of peripheral pain receptors.[97] The total salicin dose should be 30−60 mg.

3.6.5 Psychogenic Headache

Psychogenic   headaches   require psychological measures, such as a reassuring talk,[96] with the phytotherapeutic agents discussed in Section 3.5 (Psychosomatic Disorders) given in addition. Two that have proved particularly useful are St. John's wort preparations (proprietary products, see p. 62) and Species nervinae pro infantibus (p. 61).

3.6.6 Migraine Attacks

For **migraine attacks** and especially their prevention in adults, a number of clinical trials with a standardized extract (see proprietary products, p. 64) of **feverfew, *Chrysanthemum parthenium* (L.) Bernhard** (syn. *Tanacetum parthenium* L.) have given positive results.[75, 76] This medicinal plant has not yet been investigated for paediatric use. Reference to the absence of undesirable side effects in the six most recent clinical trials (1981−1988) suggested that paediatric use may be justifiable, within limits. The action is thought to be due to inhibition of serotonin release.

Apart from the **ergot alkaloids** used in the treatment of adults, no other suitable medicinal plants or natural substances are known in phytotherapy. It is interesting to note that Wiesenauer also makes no reference to medication suitable for migraine in children in his homoeopathic practice manual for paediatricians.[98]

3.6.7 Proprietary Products

a) **Tension headache**
   Various mint oils, menthol sticks, Grünlich Hingfong® solution, balm cordials, Olbas drops
b) **Pain in extremities**
   Phytodolor® N drops, Salus Schmerzetten® coated tablets, Zeller Kopfschmerz (headache) tablets, Rheumacaps capsules.
c) Migraine headaches
   Partenelle® capsules (registered in Switzerland)

3.7 Phytotherapy in the Treatment of Poisoning

Children in the Federal German Republic will take something "that does not agree with them" about 100,000 times a year.[67] 10% of these are "genuine" cases of serious poisoning, about 90% of them unfortunately fatal. It is not uncommon for the child's condition to be made worse by inexperienced treatment.

3.7.1 Emetics

One of the wrong things to do is to give saline as an emetic. If the child fails to vomit, life-threatening **hypernatraemia** may develop. A teaspoonful of salt can be fatal to an infant, a tablespoonful to a 3-year-old.

Sirupus Ipecacuanhae is a far less dangerous alternative. It consists of

Ipecacuanhae tinctura *Ger. P.* 10	1 part
Sirupus simplex	9 parts

(Note: This is the "old" formula from *Ger. P.* 6, using the ipecacuanha tincture from *Ger. P.* 10.)

Another formula [70] is the following:

Extr. Ipecacuanhae fluidum	7.0
Glycerinum	10.0
Sirupus simplex	ad 100.0

The **ipecacuanha syrup** doses recommended by toxicologists are

10 ml at age 1 – 1½ years
15 ml at age 1½ – 2 years
20 ml at age 2 – 3 years
30 ml at above 3 years of age

If there are children in the house, ipecacuanha syrup should be part of the family medicine chest. It has to be remembered, however, that its shelf-life of about 1 year applies only if stored at not more than 5 °C. In many countries ipecacuanha syrup is a prescription-only medicine (pom).

If plenty of water is taken in addition, the stomach will empty more effectively. About 15 minutes later, give **charcoal**, e.g. **Coffeae carbo**, and 30 minutes after that – unless a physician has taken over – Glauber's salt (sodium sulphate).

Use of emetics is contraindicated if the patient is unconscious or if tensides have been taken, as this may cause asphyxiation. For different reasons vomiting also should not be induced if corrosive substances have been taken. In that case, lavage with and drinking of **linseed mucilage** is the method of choice. Put about 3 tablespoons of coarsely ground linseed into 1 litre of cold water and heat for about 10 minutes on a low flame, stirring all the time. When cooled to about 30 °C strain through a muslin cloth (or gauze bandage).

In conclusion, attention is drawn to information available on a 24-hour basis from poison centres. In English-speaking countries the address and telephone number of your nearest poison centre may be obtained from the local pharmacy or hospital.

3.7.2 Poison Centres

Poison Centres usually provide an 24 hours telephone information service in cases of acute poisonings. In the following a selection of poison centres in Germany, the UK and the USA is given.

Germany

Beratungsstelle für Vergiftungserscheinungen und Embryonaltoxikologie (ITOX im BBGes), Pulsstraße 3–7, 14059 **Berlin**, Tel: 0 30/1 92 40

Informationszentrale gegen Vergiftungen, Zentrum für Kinderheilkunde der Rheinischen Friedrich-Wilhelms-Universität Bonn, Adenauerallee 119, 53113 **Bonn**, Tel: 02 28/2 87-32 11 und 02 28/2 87-33 33

Universitätsklinik Freiburg, Informationszentrale für Vergiftungen, Mathildenstr. 1, 79106 **Freiburg**, Tel: 07 61/2 70-43 61

Giftinformationszentrum (GIZ)-Nord, Zentrum für Pharmakologie und Toxikologie, Robert-Koch-Straße 40, 37075 **Göttingen**, Tel: 0 5 51/1 92 40 und 05 51/38 31 80

Universitätskliniken, Kliniken für Kinder- und Jugendmedizin, Informations- und Beratungszentrum für Vergiftungen, 66421 **Homburg/Saar**, Tel: 0 68 41/1 92 40

United Kingdom

National Poisons Information Service, New Cross Hospital, Avonley Road, **London** SE14 5ER, Tel: 0 171 635 9191

National Poisons Information Service (Birmingham Centre), City Hospital NHS Trust, Dudley Road, Winson Green, **Birmingham** B18 7QH, Tel: 0 121 5 07 5 588/9

Yorkshire Regional Drug & Poisons Information Service-Leeds, The General Infirmary, Great George Street, **Leeds** LS1 3EX, Tel: 01 132 430 715; 01 132 923 547

Northern Regional Drug and Therapeutics Centre, Wolfson Unit, Claremont Place, **Newcastle** upon Tyne NE1 4LP, Tel: 0 191 2 325 131

National Poisons Information Service (Edinburgh), Scottish Poisons Information Bureau, The Royal Infirmary, 1 Lauriston Place, **Edinburgh** EH3 9YW, Tel: 0 131 5 362 300

Welsh National Poisons Unit, Ward West 5, Llandough Hospital, Penarth, South Glamorgan CF64 2XX, **Cardiff**, Tel: 01 222 709 901

Royal Group of Hospitals, Poisons Information Centre, Grosvenor Road **Belfast** B12 6BA, Tel: 0 1 232 240 503

United States of America

Alabama
Regional Poison Control Center, The Children's Hospital of Alabama, 1600-7th Avenue South, **Birmingham**, AL 35233-1711. Tel: 205/939-9201; 800/292-6678 (AL only); 205/933-4050.

Arizona
Arizona Poison and Drug Information Center, Arizona Health Sciences Center, Rm. 1156, 1501 North Campbell Avenue, **Tucson**, AZ 85724. Tel: 800/362-0101 (AZ only); 520/626-6016.

California
Central California Regional Poison Control Center, Valley Children's Hospital, 3151 N. Millbrook, IN31, **Fresno**, CA 93703. Tel: 800/346-5922 (Central CA only); 209/445-1222. San Diego Regional Poison Center, UCSD Medical Center, 200 West Arbor Drive, **San Diego**, CA 92103-8925.

Tel: 619/534-6000; 800/876-4766 (A only). San Francisco Bay Area Regional Poison Control Center, San Francisco General Hospital, 1001 Potrero Ave., Building 80, Room 230, **San Francisco**, CA 94110. Tel: 800/523-2222.

Colorado
Rocky Mountain Poison and Drug Center, 8802 E. 9th Avenue, **Denver**, CO 80220-6800. Tel: 303/629-1123.

District of Columbia
National Capital Poison Center, 3201 New Mexico Ave. NW, Suite 310, **Washington**, DC 20016. Tel: 202/625-3333; 202/362-8563 (TTY).

Florida
The Florida Poison Information Center and Toxicology Resource Center, Tampa General Hospital, **Tampa**, FL 33601. Tel: 813/253-4444 (Tampa); 800/282-3171 (Florida).

Georgia
Georgia Poison Center, Hughes Spalding Children's Hospital Grady Health Systems, 80 Butler Street S.E., **Atlanta**, GA 30335-3801. Tel: 800/282-5846 (GA only); 404/616-9000.

Indiana
Indiana Poison Center, Methodist Hospital of Indiana, I-65 & 21st Street, **Indianapolis**, IN 46206-1367. Tel: 800/382-9097 (IN only); 317/929-2323.

Maryland
Maryland Poison Center, University of Maryland School of Pharmacy, 20 North Pine Street, **Baltimore**, MD 21201. Tel: 410/706-7701; 800/492-2414 (MD only). National Capital Poison Center (D.C. suburbs only), 3201 New Mexico Ave. NW, Suite 310, **Washington**, DC 20016. Tel: 202/625-3333; 202/362-8563 (TTY).

Massachusetts
Massachusetts Poison Control System, The Children's Hospital, 300 Longwood Avenue, **Boston**, MA 02115. Tel: 617/232-2120; 800/682-9211.

Michigan
Poison Control Center, Children's Hospital of Michigan, Harpers Professional Office Building, 4160 John R. Suite 425, **Detroit**, MI 48201.
Tel: 313/745-5711.

Minnesota
Minnesota Regional Poison Center, 8100 34th Avenue S., **Minneapolis**, MN 55440–1309.
Tel: 612/221-2113.

Missouri
Cardinal Glennon Children's Hospital, Regional Poison Center, 1465 South Grand Blvd., **St. Louis**, MO 63104.
Tel: 314/772-5200; 800/366-8888.

Montana
Rocky Mountain Poison and Drug Center, 8802 E. 9th Avenue, **Denver**, CO 80220-6800.
Tel: 303/629-1123.

Nebraska
The Poison Center, 8301 Dodge Street, **Omaha**, NE 68114.
Tel: 402/390-5555 (Omaha); 800/955-9119 (NE & WY).

New Jersey
New Jersey Poison Information and Education System, 201 Lyons Avenue, **Newark**, NJ 07112.
Tel: 800/764-7661 (NJ).

New Mexico
New Mexico Poison and Drug Information Center, University of New Mexico, Health Science Libary, Room 125, **Albuquerque**, NM 87131-1076.
Tel: 505/843-2551; 800/432-6866 (NM only).

New York
New York City Poison Control Center, N.Y.C. Department of Health, 455 First Avenue, Room 123, **New York**, NY 10016.
Tel: 212/340-4494; 212/P-O-I-S-O-N-S; 212/689-9014 (TDD).

North Carolina
Carolinas Poison Center
Carolinas Medical Center, 1012 S. Kings Drive 206
Charlotte, NC 28232-2861
Tel: 704/355 4000; 800/84-TOXIN (1-800-848-6946)

Ohio
Central Ohio Poison Center, 700 Children's Drive, **Columbus**, OH 43205-2696.
Tel: 614/228-1323; 800/682-7625; 614/228-2272 (TTY).

Oregon
Oregon Poison Center, Oregon Health Sciences University, 3181 SW Sam Jackson Park Road, CB 550, **Portland**, OR 97201.
Tel: 503/494-8968; 800/452-7165 (OR only).

Pennsylvania
The Poison Control Center serving the greater Philadelphia metropolitan area, 3600 Sciences Center, Suite 220, **Philadelphia**, PA 19104-2641.
Tel: 215/386-2100.

Rhode Island
Rhode Island Poison Center, 593 Eddy Street, **Providence**, RI 02903.
Tel: 401/444-5727.

Texas
Southeast Texas Poison Control Center, The University of Texas, Medical Branch, 301 University Avenue, **Galveston**, TX 77555-1175.
Tel: 409/765-1420 (Galveston); 800/764-7661 (TX only). (Houston)

Utah
Utah Poison Control Center, 410 Chipeta Way, Suite 230, **Salt Lake City**, UT 84108.
Tel: 801/581-2151; 800/456-7707 (UT only).

Virginia
Blue Ridge Poison Center, University of Virginia, Health Sciences Center **Charlottesville**, VA 22901.
Tel: 804/924-5543; 800/451-1428 (VA only).

West Virginia
West Virginia Poison Center,
3110 MacCorkle Ave. S. E.
Charleston WV 25304
Tel: 800/642-3625 (WV only),
304/348-4211.

Wyoming
The Poison Center, 8301 Dodge Street,
Omaha, NE 68114.
Tel: 402/390-5555 (Omaha); 800/955-9119
(NE, ID, IA, KS, MO, SD).

Chapter 4
References

[1] Weiss RF. *Lehrbuch der Phytotherapie* 7th edn. Stuttgart: Hippokrates 1991.Translation of the 6th edition of the same: *Herbal Medicine*. English by A.R. Meuss. Gothenburg: Arcanum, Beaconsfield: Beaconsfield 1985.

[2] Braun, H. and Frohne, D.: Heilpflanzen-Lexikon für Ärzte und Apotheker. 5th ed., Stuttgart: Gustav Fischer Verlag 1987.

[3] Hänsel, R. and Haas, H.: Therapie mit Phytopharmaka. Berlin-Heidelberg-New York: Springer-Verlag 1983.

[4] Reuter, H. D., Deininger, R. and Schulz, V.: Phytotherapie-Grundlagen, Klinik, Praxis. Stuttgart: Hippokrates Verlag 1987.

[5] Schimmel, K. Ch.: Lehrbuch der Naturheilverfahren. Vol.1 and Vol.2. Stuttgart: Hippokrates Verlag 1990 and 1987.

[6] Rothschuh, K. E.: Naturheilbewegung, Reformbewegung, Alternativbewegung. Stuttgart: Hippokrates Verlag 1983.

[7] Liebau, K. F.: Handbuch für die Naturheilkunde. München: Pflaum Verlag 1988

[8] Zeitschrift für Phytotherapie. Stuttgart: Hippokrates Verlag.

[9] Planta medica. Stuttgart: Thieme Verlag.

[10] Ärztezeitschrift für Naturheilverfahren. Uelzen: Medizinisch Literarische Verlagsgesellschaft mbH.

[11] Natura – med. Ärztezeitschrift mit biologischen Therapien. Mainz: Natura – med Verlagsgesellschaft mbH.

[12] Phytotherapy Research. London: Heyden & Son.

[13] Fintelmann, V.: Zukunftsaspekte der Phytotherapie. Ztsch. für Phytotherapie 8, 97−101 (1987).

[14] Hänsel, R.: Möglichkeiten und Grenzen pflanzlicher Arzneimittel (Phytotherapie). Dtsch. Apoth. Ztg. 127, 2−6 (1987).

[15] Schilcher, H.: Grundlagen, Möglichkeiten und Grenzen der Naturheilverfahren – Phytotherapie. Ärztezeitschrift f. Naturheilverfahren 29, 767−776 (1988).

[16] Vogel, G.: Rationale Therapie – Keine Chance für Heilpflanzen?. Bild der Wissenschaft No. 5, 76−88 (1981).

[17] Weiss, R. F.: Ideologische und praktische Grundlage der Naturheilkunde. Ärztezeitschrift f. Naturheilverfahren 22, 85−93 (1981).

[18] Referiert in Apotheker Zeitung 5, Heft 19, 2 (1989).

[19] Treben, M.: Gesundheit aus der Apotheke Gottes. Steyr: Wilhelm Ennsthaler 1986.

[20] Buchborn, E.: Ärztliche Erfahrung und Theorie der Heilkunde in: Beobachtung, Experiment und Theorie in Naturwissenschaft und Medizin. Verhandlungen der Ges. Dt. Naturforscher und Ärzte, 114. Versammlung, Stuttgart: Wissenschaftliche Verlagsgesellschaft mbH 1987.

[21] Bundesminister für Forschung und Technologie (Hrsg.): Forschung und Entwicklung im Dienste der Gesundheit. Bonn 1988, p. 35.

[22] Steinegger, E. and Hänsel, R.: Lehrbuch der Pharmakognosie und Phytopharmazie. Ed. R. Hänsel, 4th ed. Berlin-Heidelberg-New York: Springer-Verlag 1988.

[23] Wichtl, M. (Ed.): Teedrogen. 2nd ed. Stuttgart: Wissenschaftliche Verlagsgesellschaft mbH 1989. Translation of the same: Herbal Drugs and Phytopharmaceuticals. Translated into English and edited by N. G. Bisset. Stuttgart: Medpharm Scientific Publishers, Boca Raton: CRC Press 1994.

[24] Schilcher, H.: Möglichkeiten und Grenzen der Phytotherapie. Ärztezeitschrift f. Naturheilverfahren 28, 942−960 (1987).

[25] Keil, G.: Phytotherapie und Medizingeschichte. 24 pages. Stuttgart: Hippokrates Verlag 1985.

[26] Hänsel, R.: Möglichkeiten und Grenzen pflanzlicher Arzneimittel in: Rationale und realistische Medizin, Hrsg. Graul, E. H., Pütter, S. and Loew, D., Medicenale XVI, Iserlohn 1986, 281−291.

[27] Werning, C. (Hrsg.): Medizin für Apotheker. Stuttgart: Wissenschaftl. Verlagsgesellschaft mbH 1987.

[28] Miething, H. and Holz, W.: Menthol und Menthon in Pfefferminztees – Ermittlung der Freisetzungskinetiken. Pharm. Ztg. 133, 16−17 (1988).

[29] Hausen, B. M.: Arnikaallergie. Hautarzt 31, 10 (1980).

[30] Willuhn, G., Röttger, P. M. and Matthiesen, U.: Helenalin- und 11 α, 13-Dihydrohelenalinester aus Blüten von Arnica montana L. Planta medica 47, 157 (1983).

[31] Willuhn, G.: Arnika-Kontaktdermatitis und die sie verursachenden Kontaktallergene. Dtsch. Apoth. Ztg. 126, 2038−2044 (1986).

[32] Borneff, J. and Graf, Z.: Gutachten über die Wirkung des Minzöles (IHP-Rödler) auf die Wundbehandlung. Mainz: Hygiene Institut der Johannes Gutenberg Universität 1971.

[33] Hausen, B. M.: Die Kamille im Spektrum der kontaktsensibilisierenden Pflanzen in Klaschka, F., Maiwald, L. and Patzelt-Wencler, R. (Eds): Wir-

kungsweise und Anwendungsformen der Kamille: Berlin: Grosse Verlag 1988, 71–73.

[34] Hausen, B. M., Busker, E. and Carle, R.: Über das Sensibilisierungsvermögen von Compositenarten. Teil VII. Experimentelle Untersuchungen mit Auszügen und Inhaltsstoffen von Chamomilla recutita (L.) Rauschert und Anthemis cotula (L.). Planta medica 50, 229–234 (1984).

[35] Weidner-Strahl, S. K. and Palasser, H.: Klinische Prüfung von Wick Vaporub® beim banalen Schnupfen von Säuglingen. Wiener med. Wschr. 129, 27 (1979).

[36] Schilcher, H.: Ätherische Öle – Wirkungen und Nebenwirkungen. Dtsch. Apoth. Ztg. 124, 1433–1442 (1984).

[37] Hamann, K. F. and Bonkowsky, V.: Minzöl-Wirkung auf die Nasenschleimhaut von Gesunden. Dtsch. Apoth. Ztg. 127, 855–858 (1987).

[38] Weyers, W. and Brodbeck, R.: Hautdurchdringung ätherischer Öle. Pharmazie in unserer Zeit 18, 82–86 (1989).

[39] Schilcher, H.: Pharmakologie und Toxikologie ätherischer Öle. Therapiewoche 36, 1100–1112 (1986).

[40] Hauschild, F. in Gildemeister, E. and Hoffmann, Fr.: Die Ätherischen Öle. Vol. 1, p. 112 ff. and further volumes. Berlin: Akademie Verlag 1956 and 1961.

[41] Goodman and Gilman's: The Pharmacological Basis of Therapeutics. 6th. ed. New York-Toronto-London: Macmillan Publishing Co. Inc. 1980.

[42] Schäfer, D. and Schäfer, W.: Nachweis der sekretolytisch-expektorierenden Wirkung von Pinimenthol bei perkutaner Anwendung. Arzneimittel-Forsch. 31, 82 (1981).

[43] Ammon, H. P. T. in: Arzneimittelneben- und Wechselwirkungen. 2nd ed. Stuttgart: Wissenschaftl. Verlagsgesellschaft 1985.

[44] Holz, W.: Aucubin und andere analytische Leitstoffe zur Prüfung der pharmazeutischen Qualität von Plantago-Arten und deren Zubereitungen. Dissertation Freie Universität Berlin (1987).

[45] Müller-Limmroth, W. and Fröhlich, H. H.: Wirkungsnachweis einiger phytotherapeutischer Expektorantien auf dem mukoziliaren Transport. Fortschritte der Medizin 98, 95–101 (1980).

[46] Husten – Hintergrundinformationen für die Empfehlung des Apothekers. Supplement 5 to Nr. 3 of Dtsch. Apoth. Ztg. January (1987).

[47] Body, E. M. and Knight, L. M.: J. Pharm. Pharmacol. 16, 118 (1964).

[48] Schilcher, H.: Anwendungsmöglichkeiten des TAS-Verfahrens bei Herba Droserae, Cumarindrogen und Arzneispezialitäten mit ätherischem Öl. Dtsch. Apoth. Ztg. 114, 181–184 (1974).

[49] Fischer, E.: Über Pertussin. Therapeutische Beilage Nr. 7, p. 49 in Dtsch. med. Wschr. Juli (1898).

[50] Saller, R., Briemann, L., Travers, S. and Bühring, M.: Häusliche Inhalation mit Lindenblüten oder heißem Wasser bei akuter Erkältungskrankheit. Poster at the 2. Wissenschaftl. Tagung der Gesellschaft für Phytotherapie, Münster, Oktober 1988, submitted for publication to Zeitschrift für Phytotherapie.

[51] Schilcher, H.: Probleme bei der Beschaffung von Drogen mit Arzneibuchqualität. Pharm. Ztg. 126, 2119–2128 (1981).

[52] Hänsel, R.: Steigerung körpereigener Abwehr: Slogan oder Realität? Apotheker Journal Heft 9, 64–71 (1986).

[53] Bauer, R. and Wagner, H.: Echinacea – Der Sonnenhut – Stand der Forschung. Zeitschr. für Phytotherapie 9, 151–159 (1988).

[54] Bauer, R., Remiger, P. Jurcic, K. and Wagner, H.: Beeinflussung der Phagozytose-Aktivität durch Echinacea-Extrakte. Zeitschr. f. Phytotherapie 10, 43–48 (1989).

[55] Rösch, W.: Reizmagen – Reizdarm – Plädoyer für eine differenzierte Therapie. Medizinische Klinik 81, 316–319 (1986).

[56] Schilcher, H.: Diuretika und Harnwegsdesinfizientia. Urologe [B] 27, 368–370 (1987).

[57] Schilcher, H.: Pflanzliche Diuretika. Urologe [B] 27, 215–222 (1987).

[58] Janssen, H., Patz, B. and Wackerle, L.: Untersuchungen zur Wirksamkeit und Verträglichkeit von Uro-Fink®. Therapiewoche 37, 709–714 (1987).

[59] BGA-Pressedienst Nr. 4/1985 dated 25. 4. 1985.

[60] Nitsch-Fritz, R., Egger, H., Wutzel, H. and Maruna, H.: Ergebnisse einer Praxisstudie über das Kürbiskern-Diätetikum Kürbis-Granufink® bei Patienten mit Miktionsbeschwerden verschiedener Genese. Ztschr. Dr. Med. Nr. 5 (1979).

[61] Schilcher, H.: Cucurbita-Species. Ztschr. für Phytotherapie 7, 19–23 (1986).

[62] Lenau, H., Höxter, G., Müller, A. and Maier-Lenz, H.: Wirksamkeit und Verträglichkeit von Cysto Fink bei Patienten mit Reizblase und/oder Harninkontinenz. Therapiewoche 34, 6054–6059 (1984).

[63] Braun, R., Dittmar, W., Machut, M. and Weickmann, S.: Valepotriate mit Epoxidstruktur – beachtliche Alkylantien. Dtsch. Apoth. Ztg. 122, 1109–1112 (1982).

[64] Dittmar, W., Braun, R., Bentien, C. and Roll, R.: Activity of Valepotriates in the NBP- und Ames-Test. Naunyn-Schmiedberg's Arch. Phar. 316, R 14 Abst. 56 (1981).

[65] Dieckmannm, H.: Untersuchungen zur Pharmakokinetik, Metabolismus und Toxikologie von Baldrinalen. Dissertation an der Freien Universität Berlin, März (1989).

[66] Wohlfart, R.: Hopfen-Mite-Sedativum oder Placebo?. Dtsch. Apoth. Ztg. 123, 1637–1638 (1983).

[67] Müller-Plettenberg, D.: Vergiftungen bei Kindern. Fortschr. Med. 1, 19 (1989), ref. in Apoth. Ztg. 5, 24. April (1989), p. 4.

[68] Schwenk, H. U. and Horbach, L.: Vergleichende klinische Untersuchungen über die Wirksamkeit von Carminativum-Hetterich® bei Kindern mittels wiederholter Sonographie des Abdomens. Therapie-Woche 28, 2610–2615 (1978).

[69] Schönhöfer, P. S., Schulte-Sasse, H. and Dress, B.: Naturheilkundliche Arzneimittel: immer wirksam und unbedenklich? Pädiatrische Praxis 39, 351–357 (1989).

[70] Schulte, F. J. and Spranger, J.: Lehrbuch der Kinderheilkunde. 26th ed. Stuttgart-New York: Gustav Fischer Verlag 1988.

[71] Hoekelmann, R. A., Blatman, S., Friedmann, St. B., Nelson, N. M. and Seidel, H. M.: Primary Pediatric care. St. Louis-Washington, DC.-Toronto: The C. V. Mosby Company 1987.

[72] Heubl, G. R. and Bauer, R.: Echinacea-Arten. Dtsch. Apoth. Ztg. 129, 2497–2499 (1989).

[73] Bauer, R. and Wagner, H.: Echinacea-Handbuch für Ärzte, Apotheker und andere Naturwissenschaftler. Stuttgart: Wissenschaftl. Verlagsgesellschaft mbH 1990.

[74] Schönhöfer, P. S. and Schulte-Sasse, H.: Über die Wirksamkeit und Unbedenklichkeit von pflanzlichen Immunstimulantien. Deutsche Medizinische Wochenschrift 114, 1804 (1989) and 115, 317 (1990).

[75] Johnson, E. S., Kadam, N. P., Hyland, D. M. and Hylands, P. J.: Die Wirksamkeit von Tanacetum parthenium bei der Prophylaxe von Migräneanfällen. British Med. J. 291, 569–573 (1985).

[76] Murphy, J. J., Heptinstall, S. and Mitchel, J. R. A.: Randomisierte Doppelblindstudie mit Tanacetum parthenium zur Migräneprophylaxe. The Lancet 189–192, 23. 7. 1988.

[77] Schilcher, H.: Kombinationspräparate in der Phytotherapie. Ärztezeitschr. für Naturheilv. 31, 88–93 (1990).

[78] Schilcher, H.: Phytotherapie und Ganzheitsmedizin. Natur- und GanzheitsMedizin 3, 78–80 (1990).

[79] Haselhuber, A., Kleinschmidt, H. and Knust von Wedel, S.: Enuresis nocturna – Erfahrungen in einer Kinderkurklinik. Hippokrates 40, No. 3, 105–106 (1969).

[80] Schmitz, B.: Monographie-Uzara. Dokumentation im Auftrag der Kooperation Phytopharmaka des BPI, BHA und VRH, 72 pages (1987).

[81] Vásquez, J. L. P.: Evaluación Clinica de Uzara en Emergencia Pediátrica. Semana médica de Mexico 56, 333 (1968).

[82] Kurth, W.: Therapeutische Wirksamkeit und Akzeptanz von Linusit®. Der Kassenarzt 16, 3546 (1976).

[83] Wölbing, R. H. and Milbradt, R.: Klinik und Therapie des Herpes simplex. Therapie Woche 34, 1193–1200 (1984).

[84] Klich, R.: Verhaltensstörungen im Kindesalter und deren Therapie. Med. Welt 26, 1251–1254 (1975).

[85] Pletz, H. D.: Sedativa und Roborantia in der Behandlung von Heimkindern aus einem Großstadtmilieu. Hippokrates 34, 446–450 (1963).

[86] Bauer, G.: Ergebnisse einer Behandlung sogenannter „schwieriger Kinder". Hippokrates 32, 454–456 (1961).

[87] Wurst, F.: Erfahrungen mit dem Sedativum Valdispert® bei Lernschwierigkeiten von Kindern. Der praktische Arzt 12, 753–757 (1958).

[88] Kirschninck, H.: Beitrag zur Frage der Wirkung von Baldrian-Dispert. Hippokrates 31, 90–92 (1960).

[89] Daniel, K. W. O.: Über die Behandlung psychosomatischer Fehlhaltungen bzw. Störungen bei Kindern im Alter zwischen 6 und 12 Jahren mit einem Vollextrakt aus Hypericum perforatum. Physik. Med. und Rehab. 15, No. 3 (1974).

[90] Hänsel, R.: Phytopharmaka – 2., völlig überarbeitete Auflage. Berlin-Heidelberg-New York: Springer-Verlag 1991.

[91] Swoboda, M. and Meurer, J.: Therapie von Neurodermitis mit Hamamelis-virginiana-Extrakt in Salbenform. Zeitschr. f. Phytotherapie 12, 114–117 (1991).

[92] Schütz, E.: Akute Diarrhö – Selbstmedikation mit Loperamid. Dtsch. Apoth. Ztg. 131, 901–902 (1991).

[93] Bunjes, R., Mühlendahl, K. E. and Krienka, E. G.: Gefahr des Ileus durch das Antidiarrhoikum Loperamid. Pädiatrische Praxis 20, (2) 217–218 (1978).

[94] Allain, R., Fleurentin, J., Lanhers, M. C., Younos, Ch., Misslin, R., Mortier, F. and Pelt, J. M.: Behavioural Effects of the American Traditional Plant Eschscholzia californica: Sedative and Anxiolytic Properties. Planta med. 57, 212–216 (1991).

[95] Römmelt, H., Schnizer, W., Swoboda, M. and Senn, E.: Pharmakokinetik ätherischer Öle nach Inhalation mit einer terpenhaltigen Salbe. Zeitschr. f. Phytotherapie 9, 14–16 (1988).

[96] Dorsch, Walter, Kinderklinik und Kinder-Poliklinik der Johannes-Gutenberg-Universität Mainz – personal communication.

[97] Meier, B. and Liebi, M.: Salicinhaltige pflanzliche Arzneimittel – Überlegungen zu Wirksamkeit und Unbedenklichkeit. Zeitschr. f. Phytotherapie 11, 50–58 (1990).

[98] Wiesenauer, M.: Pädiatrische Praxis der Homöopathie. Stuttgart: Hippokrates Verlag 1989.

[99] Stopfkuchen, H.: Notfälle im Kindesalter – Außerklinische Erstversorgungsmaßnahmen. Stuttgart: Wissenschaftliche Verlagsgesellschaft mbH 1992.

[100] Von Harnack, G. A. and Jansen, F.: Pädiatrische Dosistabellen. Stuttgart: Wissenschaftliche Verlagsgesellschaft mbH 1992.

[101] Schimmel, K. Ch.: Phytotherapie im Kindesalter. Ärztezeitschr. f. Naturheilverf. 32, 137–142 (1991).

[102] McFarland LV, Bernasconi P. Saccharomyces Boulardii – A Review of an Innovative Biotherapeutic Agent. *Microbial Ecology in Health and Disease* vol. 6, pp. 157–171. 1993.

[103] Chapoy P. Traitement des diarrhées aigues infantiles. Essay controlé de Saccharomyces Boulardii. *Annales de Pédiatrie* 1985; **32**: 61–3.

[104] Schilcher H. Plant alternatives to benzodiapines and other chemoagents. *54th International Congress of Federation International Pharmaceutique (FIP)*. Lisbon, Portugal, 4-9 September 1994. Dtsch. Apoth. Ztg., Heft Nr. 20 (1995).

[105] Dorsch W, Loew D, Meyer E, Schilcher H. *Empfehlungen zu Kinderdosierungen von monographischen Arzneidrogen und ihren Zubereitungen.* Kooperation Phytopharmaka, Bonn 1993. ISBN 3-929964-11-2.

[106] Buchbauer, G., Jirovetz, L., Jäger, W., Dietrich, H., Plank, Ch., Karamat, E.: Aromatherapy: Evidence for Sedative Effects of the Essential Oil of Lavender after Inhalation. Z. Naturforsch. 46c, 1067–1072 (1991).

Chapter 5
Commission E Monographs

**(Commission for the registration and preparation of drugs
in the sphere of human medicine, phytotherapeutic
medicine and substances, at the former Federal German Department
of Health, Berlin = BGA)**

5.1 Introduction to the Monographs

This chapter gives the Commission E Monographs (published in the Federal Gazette or in draft form in specialist journals for public discussion) of all the phytomedicines referred to in this book. The monographs are in alphabetical order. Commission E is an interdisciplinary expert body appointed by the former Department of Health at the Federal German Department of Health every three years. As a commission responsible for registration and preparation of drugs in the sphere of human medicine,

(phytomedicines and substances), its function is to process scientific data on medicinal plants and herbal preparations to produce monographs.

Concerning the indications given in the monographs, it should be noted that in the majority of cases, only a few indications out of the wide spectrum of actions known in empirical medicine have been properly documented and can therefore be accepted as scientific. For this reason, only a limited number of the indications listed in the "lyrical" works of popular medicine have found their way into the monographs. The Posology refers to use for adults. The posology normally used in paediatrics, i.e. dose per body surface (m^2) or per body weight (kg), is not included in the monographs.

A rough guide for dosage of phytotherapeutic drugs is ⅓ **of the adult dose** given in the monograph for very young and young children and ½ **the adult dose for schoolchildren**.

A table of paediatric doses of the kind available for synthetic drugs [100] exists only for 75 herbal drugs [105].

5.2 Alphabetical List of Monographs
(International Latin Terms)

Absinthii herba
Achillea millefolium
Adonidis herba
Aloe
Althaeae folium
Althaeae radix
Angelicae fructus/herba
Angelicae radix
Anisi fructus
Arnicae flos
Aurantii pericarpium
Avenae herba
Avenae stramentum
Balsamum peruvianum
Balsamum tolutanum
Betulae folium
Bursae pastoris herba
Calendulae flos
Camphora
Carvi aetheroleum
Carvi fructus
Caryophylli flos
Centaurii herba
Coffeae carbo
Colchicum autumnale
Condurango cortex
Crataegi folium cum flore
Cucurbitae peponis semen
Droserae herba
Echinaceae purpureae herba
Equiseti herba
Eschscholtzia californica
Eucalypti aetheroleum
Eucalypti folium
Euphrasiae herba
Farfarae flos/-herba/-radix
Farfarae folium
Filipendula ulmaria
Foeniculi fructus
Frangulae cortex
Galeopsidis herba
Gentianae radix
Hamamelidis folium et cortex

Hederae helicis folium
Hippocastani semen
Hyperici herba
Lavandulae flos
Ledi palustris herba
Lichen islandicus
Lini semen
Liquiritiae radix
Lupuli strobulus
Malvae flos
Malvae folium
Mate folium
Matricariae flos
Melissae folium
Menthae arvensis aetheroleum
Menthae piperitae aetheroleum
Menthae piperitae folium
Myrrha
Myrtilli folium
Myrtilli fructus
Ononidis radix
Origani vulgaris herba
Orthosiphonis folium
Passiflorae herba
Piceae turiones recentes
Pini aetheroleum
Pini turiones
Plantaginis lanceolatae herba
Pollen
Polygalae radix
Primulae flos
Primulae radix
Psyllii semen
Raphani sativi radix
Rhei radix
Salicis cortex
Salviae folium
Sambuci flos
Senna
Serpylli herba
Solidago
Symphyti radix
Syzygii cumini cortex

Taraxaci radix cum herba
Terebinthinae aetheroleum rectificatum
Terebinthinae Laricina
Thymi herba
Tiliae flos
Tiliae folium
Tormentillae rhizoma

Usnea species
Uvae ursi folium
Uzarae radix
Valerianae radix
Verbasci flos
Violae tricoloris herba
Zingiberis rhizoma

5.3 Alphabetical List of Indications given in the Commission E Monographs

Indications	Monographs
Anal and genital region, diseases of	Matricariae flos
Anxiety states	Hyperici herba Lupuli strobulus
Appetite, loss of	Absinthii herba Achillea millefolium Angelicae radix Aurantii pericarpium Centaurii herba Condurango cortex Gentianae radix Lichen islandicus Pollen Taraxaci radix cum herba
Bedsores	Balsamum peruvianum
Bile ducts, dyskinesia	Absinthii herba Raphani sativi radix
Biliary flow, disorders	Taraxaci radix cum herba
Bladder outlet obstruction with prostatic adenoma stages I and II	Cucurbitae peponis semen
Bladder, irritable	Cucurbitae peponis semen
Boils	Terebinthinae laricina
Bronchial disease, chronic	Hederae helicis folium Terebinthinae aetheroleum rectificatum
Brucellosis (Malta fever), familial	Colchicum autumnale
Bruises	Arnicae flos Symphyti radix
Burns	Balsamum peruvianum Hyperici herba

Indications	Monographs
Cardiac output progressively reduced	Crataegi folium cum flore
Cardiac symptoms	Camphora
Cardiac output reduced, esp. with nervous or anxiety symptoms present	Adonidis herba
Cardiovascular disorders	Camphora Lavandulae flos
Catarrhal conditions of respiratory tract	Anisi fructus Balsmum tolutanum Camphora Eucalypti aetheroleum Eucalypti folium Farfarae folium Galeopsidis herba Hederae helicis folium Liquiritiae radix Matricariae flos Menthae arvensis aetheroleum Menthae piperitae aetheroleum Piceae turiones recentes Pini aetheroleum Pini turiones Plantaginis lanceolatae herba Primulae flos Raphani sativi radix Serpylli herba Terebinthinae laricina Thymi herba Verbasci flos
Colds	Filipendula ulmaria Sambuci flos
Colicky pain in gastrointestinal region	Achillea millefolium Angelicae radix Carvi aetheroleum Carvi fructus Foeniculi fructus Matricariae flos Menthae piperitae aetheroleum Menthae piperitae folium
Colon damaged by laxative abuse	Lini semen

Indications	Monographs
Colon, irritable	Lini semen Menthae piperitae aetheroleum Psylii semen
Conditions where ease of defecation with soft stools is desirable, e.g. anal fissures, haemorrhoids, after anorectal surgery	Aloes Frangulae cortex Rhei radix Sennae folium or Sennae fructus
Conjunctivitis simplex	Euphrasia herba
Constipation	Aloes Frangulae cortex Rhei radix Sennae folium or Sennae fructus
Constipation, chronic habitual	Lini semen Psyllii semen
Contusions	Arnicae flos Symphyti radix
Cough, paroxysmal	Droserae herba
Cramps, leg, night-time	Hippocastani semen
Dental conditions (local pain relief)	Caryophylli flos
Depressive states	Hyperici herba
Diverticulitis	Lini semen
Dry, irritant cough	Althaeae folium Althaeae radix Droserae herba Lichen islandicus Malvae flos Malvae folium
Enteritis	Lini semen
Epigastric symptoms, functional	Lavandulae flos Melissae folium Menthae arvensis aetheroleum
Epistaxis	Bursae pastoris herba
Exhaustion (mental and physical)	Mate folium
Febrile conditions	Salicis cortex

Indications	Monographs
Flatulence	Angelicae radix Carvi aetheroleum Carvi fructus Foeniculi fructus Gentianae radix Lavandulae flos Menthae arvensis aetheroleum
Fracture oedema	Arnicae flos
Frostbite, chilblains	Balsamum peruvianum
Furunculosis following insect bites	Arnicae flos
Gastritis	Lini semen
Gastritis and enteritis	Rhei radix
Gastritis (mild)	Althaeae radix
"Geriatric" heart, not requiring digitalization	Crataegi folium cum flore
Gout (acute attack)	Colchicum autumnale
Haematoma	Arnicae flos
Haemorrhoids	Balsamum peruvianum Hamamelidis folium et cortex
Headache	Salicis cortex
Heart region, sensation of pressure and oppression	Crataegi folium cum flore
Indigestion	Absinthii herba Achillea millefolium Angelicae radix Anisi fructus Aurantii pericarpium Carvi aetheroleum Carvi fructus Centaurii herba Foeniculi fructus Hyperici herba Salviae folium Taraxaci radix cum herba Zingiberis rhizoma

Indications	Monographs
Infections (recurrent) in respiratory and lower urinary tract	Echinaceae purpureae herba
Inflammation caused by insect bites	Arnicae flos, Caryophylli aetheroleum
Inflammation (local)	Lini semen
Inflammation of oral and pharyngeal mucosa	Arnicae flos Calendulae flos Caryophylli flos Coffeae carbo Farfarae folium Matricariae flos Menthae piperitae aetheroleum Myrrha Myrtilli fructus Plantaginis lanceolatae herba Salvia folium Syzygii cumini cortex Tormentillae rhizoma
Inflammation of respiratory tract	Matricariae flos
Inflammatory conditions in gastrointestinal region	Matricariae flos
Inflammatory conditions of lower urinary tract	Uvae ursi folium
Inflammatory skin conditions	Avenae stramentum Hamamelidis folium et cortex Matricariae flos Plantaginis lanceolatae herba Syzygii cumini cortex
Intestines, clearing prior to operations or X-rays	Sennae folium or Sennae fructus
Irrigation treatment for inflammatory conditions of lower urinary tract, renal sand or gravel	Betulae folium Equiseti herba Ononidis radix Orthosiphonis folium Solidaginis herba Taraxaci radix cum herba Uvae ursi folium
Meteorism	Lavandulae flos Menthae arvensis aetheroleum

Indications	Monographs
Milk crust of children	Violae tricoloris herba
Muscle and tendon strains	Symphyti radix
Muscular and nerve pain	Menthae piperitae aetheroleum Piceae turiones recentes Pini turiones
Myalgia	Hyperici herba Menthae arvensis aetheroleum
Neuralgiform pain	Menthae arvensis aetheroleum
Oedema, posttraumatic and static (I)	Equiseti herba
Pressure sores from prostheses	Balsamum peruvianum
Psychovegetative disorders	Hyperici herba
Respiratory tract irritation	Matricariae flos Usnea species
Restlessness	Lavandulae flos Lupuli strobulus Valerianae radix
Restlessness, nervous	Hyperici herba Passiflorae herba
Rheumatic complaints	Arnicae flos Betulae folium Camphora Eucalypti aetheroleum Salicis cortex
Rheumatic and neuralgic pain	Pini aetheroleum Terebinthinae aetheroleum rectificatum Terebinthinae laricina
Roborant for states of exhaustion	Pollen
Sensation of fullness	Angelicae radix Carvi aetheroleum Carvi fructus Foeniculi fructus Gentianae radix
Skin conditions (bacterial)	Matricariae flos

Indications	Monographs
Skin conditions (inflammatory and seborrhoeic, esp. with pruritus)	Avenae stramentum
Skin conditons (mild seborrhoeic)	Violae tricoloris herba
Skin conditions (inflammatory)	Matricariae flos
Sleep disorders	Lupuli strobulus
Sleep, problems going to	Lavandulae flos Melissae folium Valerianae radix
Sprains	Arnicae flos Symphyti radix
Sweating, increased	Salvia folium
Symptoms of chronic venous insufficiency, e.g. oedema, leg cramps, pruritus, pain and heaviness in legs, varicosis, postthrombotic syndrome	Hippocastani semen Rusci aculeati rhizoma
Travel sickness, prevention	Zingiberis rhizoma
Ulcer, leg (Ulcus cruris)	Balsamum peruvianum Calendulae flos Hippocastani semen
Ulcer, peptic (Ulcus ventriculi/duodeni)	Liquiritiae radix
Varicose veins, symptoms from	Hamemelidis folium et cortex
Veins, leg, chronic insufficiency	Hippocastani semen
Whooping cough	Thymi herba Droserae herba
Wounds (healing)	Balsamum peruvianum Bursae pastoris herba Calendulae flos Echinaceae purpureae herba Equiseti herba Hamamelidis folium et cortex Hyperici herba

5.4 Alphabetical List of Medicinal Actions

Actions	Monographs
Accelerated healing of gastric ulcers, acc. to clinical trials	Liquiritiae radix
Adsorbent	Coffeae carbo
Anaerobic threshold raised	Crataegi folium cum flore
Analeptic	Mate folium
Analgesic	Salicis cortex
Antibacterial	Achillea millefolium Anisi fructus Balsamum peruvianum Matricariae flos Menthae arvensis aetheroleum Menthae piperitae aetheroleum Plantaginis lanceolatae herba Salviae folium Thymi herba Uvae ursi folium
Antichemotactic	Colchicum autumnale
Antidepressant	Hyperici herba
Antiemetic	Zingiberis rhizoma
Antiexudative	Hippocastani semen
Antiflatulent	Lavandulae flos
Antiinflammatory	Arnicae flos Colchicum autumnale Ledi palustris herba Matricariae flos Salicis cortex Solidago Hyperici herba Calendulae flos Hamamelidis folium et cortex Symphyti radix Violae tricoloris herba

Actions	Monographs
Antimicrobial	Carvi aetheroleum Carvi fructus Lichen islandicus Raphani sativi radix Serpylli herba Usnea species
Antimitotic	Symphyti radix
Antiparasitic (esp. itch mite)	Balsamum peruvianum
Antipyretic	Salicis cortex
Antiseptic	Arnicae flos Balsamum peruvianum Terebinthinae aetheroleum rectificatum Terebinthinae laricina Piceae turiones recentes Pini aetheroleum Pini turiones
Antisudorific	Salviae folium
Antitussive	Droserae herba Ledi palustris herba
Aperitive	Aurantii pericarpium Condurango cortex Lichen islandicus Pollen Taraxaci radix cum herba
Astringent	Achillea millefolium Coffeae carbo Galeopsidis herba Hamamelidis folium et cortex Myrrha Myrtilli fructus Plantaginis lanceolatae herba Salviae folium Tormentillae rhizoma
Bacterial toxin inhibitor	Matricariae flos
Bacteriostatic (in alkaline [pH 8] urine)	Uvae ursi folium
Bathmotropic, negative	Crataegi folium cum flore

Actions	Monographs
Bronchial secretion increasing	Sambuci flos
Bronchial secretion reduced	Terebinthinae aetheroleum rectificatum
Bronchospasmolytic	Camphora Droserae herba Thymi herba
Bronchosecretolytic	Camphora
Callus development promoting	Symphyti radix
Cardiovascular tonic	Camphora
Carminative	Melissae folium Menthae arvensis aetheroleum Menthae piperitae aetheroleum Menthae piperitae folium
Cholagogue	Menthae arvensis aetheroleum Menthae piperitae aetheroleum Zingiberis rhizoma
Choleretic	Achillea millefolium Menthae piperitae folium Taraxaci radix cum herba
Chronotropic, negative	Crataegi folium cum flore
Chronotropic, positive	Mate folium
Cooling	Menthae arvensis aetheroleum Menthae piperitae aetheroleum
Coronary and myocardial blood supply increased	Crataegi folium cum flore
Demulcent	Altheae folium Altheae radix Lichen islandicus Malvae flos Malvae folium Verbasci flos
Deodorant	Matricariae flos

Actions	Monographs
Diuretic	Betulae folium Equiseti herba Mate folium Orthosiphonis folium Solidago Taraxaci radix cum herba
Dromotropic, negative	Crataegi folium cum flore
Dromotropic, positive	Crataegi folium cum flore
Emollient	Plantaginis lanceolatae herba
Expectorant	Anisi fructus Eucalypti aetheroleum Eucalypti folium Foeniculi fructus Hederae helicis folium Liquiritiae radix Polygalae radix Primulae flos Primulae radix Thymi herba Verbasci flos
Fungistatic	Salviae folium
Gastric fluid secretion increased	Centaurii herba Condurango cortex
Gastrointestinal motility improved	Foeniculi fructus
Glycogenolytic	Mate folium
Granulation promoting	Balsamum peruvianum
Hypnogenic	Lupuli strobulus Valerianae radix
Hypnotic	Valerianae radix
Immunobiological action in humans and in animal experiments	Echinaceae purpureae herba
Inducing active secretion of electrolytes and water into intestinal lumen and inhibiting resorption from colon	Aloe Frangulae cortex Rhei radix

Actions	Monographs
Inotropic, positive	Adonidis herba Bursae pastoris herba Crataegi folium cum flore Mate folium Zingiberis rhizoma
Intestinal tone and peristalsis increased	Zingiberis rhizoma
Laxative as bulking agent triggering peristalsis via dilatation reflex	Lini semen Psyllii semen
Laxative	Aloes and other anthranoid drugs
Lipolytic	Mate folium
Local styptic	Hamamelidis folium et cortex
Lysosomal enzyme activity, excessive, reduced	Hippocastani semen
MAO inhibitor	Hyperici herba
Mitosis inhibitor	Colchicum autumnale
Motility inhibitor	Passiflorae herba Ledi palustris herba
Motility stimulant	Raphani sativi radix
Mucociliary activity inhibiting	Althaeae radix
Mucosa protected by covering action	Lini semen
Muscarine-type actions with dose-dependent hypo-/hypertensive effect (parenteral only)	Bursae pastoris herba
Peristalsis increased to raise internal pressure; overstimulation of propulsive contractions	Aloe and other anthranoid drugs
Phagocytosis activated in human granulocytes	Echinaceae purpureae herba
Phagocytosis increasing	Altheae radix Echinaceae purpureae herba
Pyretogenic	Echinaceae purpureae herba
Respiratory analeptic	Camphora

Actions	Monographs
Rubefacient	Camphora Eucalypti aetheroleum Piceae turiones recentes Pini aetheroleum Terebinthinae aetheroleum rectificatum Terebinthinae laricina
Salivant	Condurango cortex
Salivary and gastric fluid secretion, reflex stimulation	Gentianae radix
Salivary and gastric fluid secretion promoting	Zingiberis rhizoma
Secretagogue	Salvia folium Raphani sativi radix
Secretolytic	Liquiritiae radix Menthae arvensis aetheroleum Menthae piperitae aetheroleum Piceae turiones recentes Pini aetheroleum Pini turiones Polygalae radix Primulae flos Primulae radix
Secretomotor	Eucalypti aetheroleum Eucalypti folium
Sedative	Lavandulae flos Lupuli strobulus Melissae folium Valerianae radix
Skin metabolism stimulated	Matricariae flos
Skin and mucosal irritant	Hederae helicis folium Ledi palustris herba
Sleeping time incr. following exhibition of barbiturates and ethanol	Ledi palustris herba

Actions	Monographs
Spasmolytic	Achillea millefolium
	Anisi fructus
	Carvi aetheroleum
	Carvi fructus
	Eucalypti aetheroleum
	Eucalypti folium
	Foeniculi fructus
	Hederae helicis folium
	Matricariae flos
	Menthae arvensis aetheroleum
	Menthae piperitae aetheroleum
	Orthosiphonis folium
	Serpylli herba
	Solidago
	Zingiberis rhizoma
Sudorific	Sambuci flos
Uterine contractility increased	Bursae pastoris herba
Vascular permeability reduced	Hippocastani semen
Venous tone increased	Adonidis herba
	Hippocastani semen
Virostatic	Salvia folium
Vulnerary	Calendulae flos
	Matricariae flos
White and splenic cell count increased	Echinaceae purpureae herba

5.5 Commission E Monographs passed or accepted at draft stage, in alphabetical sequence
(360 monographs processed by August 1995)

Abbreviation Banz = *Bundesanzeiger*
(Federal Gazette)

Absinthii herba
(Wormwood herb)

Banz No. 228 of 5 Dec. 1984

Official Name
Absinthii herba, wormwood herb

Description
Wormwood herb, consisting of fresh or dried upper shoots and foliage leaves collected at flowering time, or of fresh or dried basal leaves, or a mixture of the above, of *Artemisia absinthium* L. and preparations of these in effective doses. The plant drug contains not less than 0.3 per cent (v/w) of volatile oil and has a bitter index of not less than 15,000. The volatile oil contains thujone; the plant drug also contains sesquiterpene lactone bitters such as absinthin, anabsinthin, artabsin, anabsin; furthermore flavones, ascorbic acid and tannins.

Indications
Loss of appetite
Indigestion
Biliary dyskinesia

Contraindications
None reported.

Side Effects
None reported.

Interactions
None reported.

Dosage
Unless otherwise prescribed,

Mean daily dose
Aqueous extract of 2−3 g of the plant drug.

Method of Application
Minced drug for infusions and decoctions; powdered drug; also extracts or tinctures, all liquid or solid presentations for oral use only.

Note
Combination with other bitters or aromatics may be indicated.
Toxic doses of thujone, an active principle in the volatile oil, may cause convulsions. The isolated volatile oil should not be used, therefore.

Medicinal Actions
The aromatic bitter action is due to the bitter principles and volatile oils.
Recent pharmacological data that might be of use are not available.

Achillea millefolium
(Yarrow)

Banz No. 22a of 1 Feb. 1990

Official Name
Millefolii herba, yarrow herb
Millefolii flos, yarrow flowers

Description
Yarrow herb, consisting of fresh or dried aerial parts of *Achillea millefolium* L. s. l. and preparations of these in effective doses.
Yarrow flowers, consisting of the dried inflorescences (terminal corymbs) of *Achillea millefolium* L. s. l. and preparations of these in effective doses.
The plant drug contains volatile oil and proazulenes.

Indications
Taken by mouth: Loss of appetite; indigestion, e.g. mild colicky pain in gastrointestinal region.
As sitzbaths: Autonomic diseases affecting the pelvic area (painful spasms of psychological, autonomic origin in the female true pelvis.

Contraindications
Hypersensitivity to yarrow and other Compositae.

Side Effects
None reported.

Interactions
None reported.

Dosage
Unless otherwise prescribed,
Mean daily dose
Taken by mouth: 4.5g of yarrow herb, 3g of yarrow flowers; 3 teaspoonfuls of fresh plant juice; preparations in equivalent amounts.
For sitzbaths: 100g of yarrow herb to 20 litres of water.

Method of Application
Minced drug for infusions and other galenical preparations for oral route and sitzbaths; fresh plant juice for oral route.

Medicinal Actions
Choleretic
Antibacterial
Astringent
Spasmolytic

```
Adonidis herba
(Yellow pheasant's eye)
Banz No. 85 of 5 May 1988
```

Official Name
Adonidis herba, pheasant's eye herb

Description
Pheasant's eye herb, consisting of dried aerial parts of *Adonis vernalis* L. collected at flowering time and preparations of these in effective doses.

The plant drug contains cardiac glycosides and flavonoids.

Indications
Minor reduction in cardiac function, especially if accompanied by nervous anxiety.

Contraindications
Treatment with digitalis glycosides.
Potassium deficiency.

Side Effects
None reported.

Interactions
Increases activity and therefore also side effects of quinidine, calcium, saluretics, laxatives and long-term glucocorticoids if given concurrently.

Dosage
Unless otherwise prescribed,
Mean daily dose: 0.6g of standardized powder (= Adonidis pulvis normatus) of the plant (*Ger. P.* 10);
Maximum single dose: 1.0g
Maximum daily dose: 3.0g
Preparations in equivalent amounts.

Method of Application
Minced drug and preparations for oral administration.

Note
Overdose causes nausea, vomiting, cardiac arrhythmias.

Medicinal Actions
Positive inotropic,
in animal experiments improved venous tone.

```
Aloe
(Aloes)
Banz No. 133 of 21 July 1993
```

Official Name
Aloe barbadensis; Barbados (Curaçao) aloes
Aloe capensis, Cape aloes

Description
Curaçao aloes, the residue obtained by evaporating the juice from the leaves of *Aloe*

barbadensis Miller and preparations of this in effective doses.

Cape aloes, the residue obtained by evaporating the juice from the leaves of a number of *Aloe* species, especially *Aloe ferox* Miller and its hybrids, and preparations of this in effective doses.

The drug contains anthranoids, mainly of the aloes emodin type.

The plant drugs must meet the requirements of the current pharmacopoeia.

Pharmacology, pharmacokinetics, toxicology

1,8-dihydroxyanthracene derivatives have laxative properties.

These are mainly due to an action on colon motility, inhibiting stationary and stimulating propulsive contractions. This results in accelerated passage and, due to the reduction in contact time, a reduction in fluid absorption. Stimulation of active chloride secretion also causes water and electrolytes to be secreted.

Systematic studies on the kinetics of aloes preparations are still outstanding, but it may be assumed that the aglycones of the drug are absorbed in the upper duodenum, Glycosides with β-glycosidic bonds are prodrugs and neither split nor absorbed in the upper gastrointestinal tract. They are degraded to aloe-emodinanthrone by bacterial enzymes in the large intestine. Aloe-emodinanthrone is the laxative metabolite. Rhein was found in the urine of humans given 86 or 200 mg of powdered aloes by mouth. Small quantities of active metabolites such als rhein pass into mother's milk, but no laxative effect has been noted in breast-fed infants. Placental passage of rhein was found to be extremely low in animal experiments.

Drug preparations have greater general toxicity than the pure glycosides, probably because of the aglycone content. An aloe extract with $c = 23\%$ of aloin and less than 0.07% of Aloe emodin and aloin showed no mutagenic action in bacterial and mammalian test systems. Aloe emodin, emodin and chrysophanol have given partly positive results. Carcinogenic properties have not been investigated.

Indications
Chronic constipation.

Contraindications
Occlusion, acute inflammatory intestinal diseases, e. g. Crohn's disease, ulcerative colitis. Appendicitis; abdominal pain of unknown origin. Children under 12. Pregnancy.

Side Effects
In isolated instances, colicky gastrointestinal symptoms. The dose needs to be reduced in such cases.

Chronic use/abuse: Loss of electrolytes, above all potassium, proteinuria and haematuria; pigmentation of intestinal mucosa (pseudomelanosis coli) which, however, is harmless and normally disappears once the drug is discontinued. Potassium loss may cause functional cardiac disorders and muscular weakness, especially if cardiac glycosides, diuretics or adrenocortical steroids are taken concurrently.

Special precautions
Stimulant laxatives should not be taken for periods of more than 1 or 2 weeks unless advised by a physician.

Use during pregnancy and lactation
Because of inadequate toxicological studies, not to be used during pregnancy and lactation.

Interactions
Chronic use/abuse may enhance the actions of cardiac glycosides and affect those of anti-arrhythmic drugs because of the potassium loss. Potassium losses may be increased by combination with thiazide diuretics, adrenocortical steroids and liquorice root.

Dosage and method of application
Powdered aloes, aqueous ethanolic dry, condensed and fluid extracts and methanolic dry extracts for oral use.

Unless otherwise prescribed, 20–30 mg of hydroxyanthracene derivatives/day, calculated as anhydrous aloin.

The correct individual dose is the lowest dose to produce soft, formed stools.

Note
The formulation should permit daily doses that are less than usual.

Overdosage
Measures to balance electrolytes and fluids.

Specific warning
Use of stimulant laxatives for more than a short period may aggravate the constipation. The preparation should only be used if changes in diet or use bulking agents do not give the desired results.

Motorists and machine operators
No negative effects known.

Note
Urine may turn red on exhibition of the drug, which is harmless.

Althaeae folium
(Marshmallow leaves)

Banz No. 43 of 2 Mar. 1989

Official Name
Althaeae folium, marshmallow leaves

Description
Marshmallow leaves consisting of dried leaves of *Althaea officinalis* L. and preparations of these in effective doses.
The plant drug contains mucilage.

Indications
Irritation of oral and pharyngeal mucosa and dry irritant cough connected with this.

Contraindications
None reported.

Side Effects
None reported.

Interactions
None reported.

Dosage
Unless otherwise prescribed,
Daily dose: 5g of the plant drug; preparations in equivalent amounts.

Method of Application
Minced drug for aqueous extracts and other galenical preparations for oral administration.

Note
Absorption of other medicaments taken concurrently may be delayed.

Medicinal Actions
Demulcent.

Althaeae radix
(Marshmallow root)

Banz No. 43 of 2 Mar. 1989

Official Name
Althaeae radix, marshmallow root

Description
Marshmallow root, consisting of dried, unpeeled or peeled roots of *Althaea officinalis* L. and preparations of these in effective doses.
The plant drug contains mucilage.

Indications
a) Irritation of oral and pharyngeal mucosa in conjunction with unproductive, dry cough
b) Mild inflammation of gastric mucosa.

Contraindications
None reported.

Side Effects
None reported.

Interactions
None reported.
Note: Absorption of other medicaments taken concurrently may be delayed.

Dosage
Unless otherwise prescribed,
Daily dose: 6g of the plant drug; preparations in equivalent amounts.
"Marshmallow syrup" single dose 10g.

Method of Application
Minced plant drug for aqueous extracts and other galenical preparations for oral administration.
Marshmallow syrup only on indication a).

Note
Marshmallow syrup:
Diabetics need to take account of sugar content (as stated by manufacturers) … % (equivalent to … carbohydrate units).

Medicinal Actions
Demulcent and emollient
Inhibition of mucociliary activity
Increased phagocytosis

Angelicae fructus
(Angelica fruit)
Angelicae herba
(Angelica herb)

Banz No. 101 of 1 Jun. 1990

Official Name
Angelicae fructus, angelica fruit
Angelicae herba, angelica herb

Description
Angelica fruit, consisting of the fruits of *Angelica archangelica* L. and preparations of these.
Angelica herb, consisting of the aerial parts of *Angelica archangelica* L. and preparations of these.

Indications
Preparations made from angelica fruit and herb are used as diuretics and sudorifics.
Efficacy on these indications has not been substantiated.

Risks
The plant drugs contain furocoumarins which make skin more photosensitive.

Evaluation
As efficacy on the above indications has not been substantiated and there is a risk involved, clinical use cannot be recommended.

Angelicae radix
(Angelica root)

Banz No. 101 of 1. Jun. 1990

Official Name
Angelicae radix, angelica root

Description
Angelica root, consisting of dried roots and rhizomes of *Angelica archangelica* L. and preparations of these in effective doses.
The plant drug contains volatile oil, coumarin and coumarin derivatives.

Indications
Loss of appetite;
symptoms of indigestion such as mild gastrointestinal spasms, sensation of fullness, flatulence.

Contraindications
None reported.

Side Effects
The furocoumarins contained in angelica root make skin more photosensitive and in conjunction with UV irradiation may cause skin irritation. Extended exposure to the sun and intensive UV irradiation should therefore be avoided whilst taking angelica root or preparations of it.

Interactions
None reported.

Dosage
Unless otherwise prescribed,

Daily dose
4.5 g of the plant drug;
1.5−3 g of the fluidextract (1:1);
1.5 g of the tincture (1:5); preparations in equivalent amounts.
10−20 drops of the volatile oil.

Method of Application
Minced plant drug and other galenical preparations for oral administration.

Note
Extended exposure to the sun and intensive UV irradiation should be avoided whilst taking angelica root preparations.

Medicinal Actions
Spasmolytic
Cholagogue
Promotes secretion of gastric fluid

Medicinal Actions
Expectorant
Mildly spasmolytic
Antibacterial

Anisi fructus
(Aniseed)

Banz No. 122 of 6. Jul. 1988

Official Name
Anisi fructus, aniseed

Description
Aniseed, consisted of dried fruits of *Pimpinella anisum* L. and preparations of these in effective doses.
The plant drug contains volatile oil.

Indications
Internal use:
indigestion.
Internal and external use:
Catarrhal conditions of respiratory tract.

Contraindications
Allergy to anise and anethole.

Side Effects
Occasional allergic skin, respiratory and gastrointestinal tract reactions.

Interactions
None reported.

Dosage
Unless otherwise prescribed,
internal use: *Mean daily dose* 3.0g of the plant drug; 0.3g of the volatile oil; preparations in equivalent amounts;
external use: Preparations containing 5–10% of the volatile oil.

Method of Application
Minced plant drug for infusions and other galenical preparations for oral administration or inhalation.

Note
External use of aniseed preparations limited to inhalation of the volatile oil.

Arnicae flos
(Arnica flowers)

Banz No. 228 of 5 Dec. 1984

Official Name
Arnicae flos, arnica flowers

Description
Arnica flowers, consisting of fresh or dried inflorescences of *Arnica montana* L. or *Arnica chamissonis* Less. subsp. *foliosa* (Nutt.) Maguiere and preparations of these in effective doses.
The plant drug contains sesquiterpene lactones of helenanolide type and 11,13-dihydrohelenalin. The drug also contains flavonoids (e.g. isoquercitin, luteolin-7-glucoside and astragalin), volatile oil (with thymol and thymol derivatives), phenylcarboxylic acids (chlorogenic acid, cynarin, caffeic acid) and coumarins (umbelliferon, scopoletin).

Indications
External use for trauma and accidents, e.g. haematoma, sprains, contusions, oedema with fractures, rheumatic conditions affecting muscles and joints, inflammation of oral and pharyngeal mucosa, boils and inflammation following insect bites; superficial thrombophlebitis.

Contraindications
Arnica allergy.

Side Effects
Extended use on damaged skin, e.g. in case of open injuries or leg ulcers, will relatively frequently cause oedematous dermatitis with vesiculation. Eczema may also develop with extended use. High concentrations may equally provoke skin reactions and vesiculation, or even necrotic changes, that are primarily toxic in origin.

Interactions
None reported.

Dosage
Unless otherwise prescribed,
Infusion: 2.0 g of the plant drug to 100 ml of water.
Tincture: for compresses: dilute to 3–10 times the volume with water.
For mouthwashes: dilute tincture to ten times the volume.
Ointments with max. 20–25 per cent of the tincture.
"Arnica oil": Extract made with 1 part of the plant drug to 5 parts of fatty vegetable oil.
Ointments with max. 15 per cent of "Arnica oil".

Method of Application
The whole, minced or powdered plant drug for infusions, liquid and semisolid formulations for external use.

Medicinal Actions
Arnica preparations – mainly for topical application – have antiinflammatory and resultant analgesic actions as well as antiseptic properties.

Aurantii pericarpium
(Bitter orange peel)

Banz No. 193a of 15 Oct. 1987

Official Name
Aurantii pericarpium, bitter orange peel

Description
Bitter orange peel, consisting of the dried outer pericarp of ripe fruits of *Citrus aurantium* L. ssp. *aurantium* (synonym *Citrus aurantium* L. ssp. *amara* Engler) and preparations of these in effective doses.
The plant drug contains volatile oil and bitter principles.

Indications
Loss of appetite
Indigestion

Contraindications
None reported.

Side Effects
Photosensitization is possible, especially in light-skinned individuals.

Interactions
None reported.

Dosage
Daily dose
Plant drug: 4–6 g
Tincture (*Ger. P.* 7): 2–3 g
Extract (*EB* 6): 2–3 g

Method of Application
Minced drug for infusions; other bitter galenicals for oral administration.

Avenae herba
(Oat herb)

Banz No. 193a of 15 Oct. 1987

Official Name
Avenae herba, oat herb

Description
Oat herb, consisting of fresh or dried aerial parts of *Avena sativa* L. collected at flowering time, and preparations of these.

Indications
Oat herb preparations are used to treat acute and chronic anxiety states, tension and states of excitement, neurasthenia and pseudoneurasthenia syndrome, skin conditions, connective tissue weakness, weak bladder and as an anabolic and roborant.
Combined with other plant drugs, oat herb preparations are also used to treat objective and subjective cardiovascular and respiratory problems, metabolic diseases and disorders, geriatric diseases and disorders, various types of anaemia, hyperthyroidism, neuralgia and neuritis; also haematomas, muscle strains, sexual disorders, tobacco abuse, seizures and as a lactagogue and as a medicament to improve performance. Efficacy on these indications has not been substantiated.

Risks
None reported.

Evaluation
As efficacy on the above indications has not been substantiated and there is a risk involved, **clinical use cannot be recommended.**

Avenae stramentum
(Oat straw)

Banz No. 193a of 15 Oct. 1987

Official Name
Avenae stramentum, oat straw

Description
Oat straw, consisting of the dried leaves and stems left after threshing of *Avena sativa* L. and preparations of these in effective doses. The plant drug contains silica.

Indications
External use: Inflammatory and seborrhoeic skin conditions, esp. with pruritus.

Contraindications
None reported.

Side Effects
None reported.

Interactions
None reported.

Dosage
Unless otherwise prescribed,
100 g of the plant drug to a full bath; preparations in equivalent amounts.

Method of Application
Minced plant drug, decoctions of the same, and other galenical preparations as bath additives.

Balsamum peruvianum
(Peru balsam)

Banz No. 173 of 18 Sep. 1986

Official Name
Balsamum peruvianum, Peru balsam

Description
Peru balsam, consisting of balsam distilled from the trunks of *Myroxylon balsamum* (L.) Harms var. *pereira* (Royle) and preparations of this in effective doses.
Peru balsam contains 30−70 per cent of a mixture of esters, mainly benzyl esters of benzoic and cinnamic acid.

Indications
External application for infected wounds with poor healing tendencies, burns, bedsores, chilblains, leg ulcers, pressure sores from prostheses, and haemorrhoids.

Contraindications
Marked allergic disposition.

Side Effects
Allergic skin reactions.

Interactions
None reported.

Dosage
Unless otherwise prescribed,
galenical preparations containing 5−20 per cent of Peru balsam; if using over large areas, not more than 10 per cent of Peru balsam.

Method of Application
Galenical preparations for external use.

Medicinal Actions
Antibacterial/antiseptic, promotes granulation, antiparasitic (esp. itch mite).

Balsamum tolutanum
(Tolu balsam)

Banz No. 173 of 18 Sep. 1986

Official Name
Balsamum tolutanum, tolu balsam

Description
Tolu balsam, consisting of balsam obtained from cuts in the trunks of *Myroxylon balsamum* (L.) var. *balsamum* Harms (synonym *M. balsamum* var. *genuinum* [Baill] Harms) purified by melting and straining and hardened, and preparations of this in effective doses.
Tolu balsam contains benzoic and cinnamic acid and their esters and volatile oil.

Indications
Catarrhal conditions of respiratory tract.

Contraindications
None reported.

Side Effects
None reported.

Interactions
None reported.

Dosage
Unless otherwise prescribed,
Mean daily dose: 0.6 g; preparations in equivalent amounts.

Method of Application
Preparations of tolu balsam for oral administration.

Betulae folium
(Birch leaves)

Banz No. 50 of 13 Mar. 1986

Official Name
Betulae folium, birch leaves

Description
Birch leaves, consisting of fresh or dried leaves of *Betula pendula* Roth (synonym *Betula verrucosa* Ehrhart), of *Betula pubescens* Ehrhart) or both species, and preparations of these in effective doses.
The plant drug contains not less than 1.3 per cent of flavonoids, calculated as hyperoside with reference to the dried drug. It also contains saponins, tannins and volatile oil.

Indications
Irrigation therapy for bacterial and inflammatory conditions of the lower urinary tract and for renal sand or gravel; adjuvant treatment of rheumatic conditions.

Contraindications
None reported.
Note
Irrigation therapy should not be given to patients with oedema due to reduced cardiac or renal function.

Side Effects
None reported.

Interactions
None reported.

Dosage
Unless otherwise prescribed,
Mean daily dose: Several times daily 2–3 g of the drug; preparations in equivalent amounts.

Method of Application
Minced drug or dry extracts for infusions; also other galenical preparations and fresh plant extracts for oral administration.

Note
Irrigation therapy:
Fluid intake must be high.

Medicinal Actions
Diuretic

Bursae pastoris herba
(Shepherd's purse herb)

Banz No. 173 of 18 Sep. 1986

Official Name
Bursae pastoris herba, shepherd's purse herb
Description
Shepherd's purse herb, consisting of the fresh or dried aerial parts of *Capsella bursa pastoris* (L.) Medicus and preparations of these in effective doses.

Indications
Internal use: symptomatic treatment of milder forms of menorrhagia and metrorrhagia; topical use for epistaxis.
External use: superficial, bleeding skin lesions.

Contraindications
None reported.

Side Effects
None reported.

Interactions
None reported.

Dosage
Unless otherwise prescribed,
Mean daily dose: 10–15 g of the drug, preparations in equivalent amounts.
Topical use: Infusion of 3–5 g of the drug in 150 ml of water. Fluidextract (*EB* 6): daily dose 5–8 g.

Method of Application
Minced drug for infusions, also other galenical preparations for oral administration and topical use.

Medicinal Actions
With parenteral use only:
Muscarine-type actions with dose-dependent hypo- or hypertensive effects, positive inotropic and chronotropic action on heart; increased uterine contractions.

tion in ointments containing $2-5$ g of the drug per 100 g.

Method of Application
Minced drug to make infusions, and other galenical preparations for topical use.

Medicinal Actions
Vulnerary
Antiinflammatory and granulation-promoting effects have been reported with topical use.

Calendulae flos
(Garden marigold flowers)

Banz No. 50 of 13 Mar. 1986

Camphora
(Camphor)

Banz No. 228 of 5 Dec. 1984

Official Name
Calendulae flos, garden marigold flowers

Description
Garden marigold flowers, consisting of the dried flower heads or dried ligulate florets of *Calendula officinalis* L. and preparations of these in effective doses.
The plant drug contains triterpene glycosides and triterpene aglycons, carotinoids and volatile oil.

Indications
Topical internal use:
Inflammatory changes in oral and pharyngeal mucosa.
External use:
Wounds, including those with poor healing tendency. Leg ulcers.

Contraindications
None reported.

Side Effects
None reported.

Interactions
None reported.

Dosage
Unless otherwise prescribed,
$1-2$ g of the drug to 1 cup of water (150 ml)
or
$1-2$ teaspoonfuls ($2-4$ ml) of the tincture to
¼–½ litres of water, or in suitable prepara-

Official Name
Camphora, camphor

Description
D(+)-Camphor obtained by steam distillation of the wood of the camphor tree, *Cinnamomum camphora* (L.) Siebold and subsequently purified by sublimation, or synthetic camphor, or a mixture of the two. Contains not less than 96.0 and not more than 101.0 per cent of bornan-2-one. Not less than one half is in form of the (1R)-isomer.

Indications
External use: Muscular rheumatism, catarrhal conditions of the respiratory tract, cardiac complaints.
Internal use: Hypotensive cardiovascular disorders, catarrhal conditions of the respiratory tract.

Contraindications
External use: Damaged skin, e.g. burns. With infants and young children, camphor-containing preparations should not be applied in the region of the face, esp. the nose.

Side Effects
Contact eczema may occur.

Interactions
None reported.

Dosage
Unless otherwise prescribed,

external use: depending on use on limited area, generally in concentrations of not more than 25 per cent, for infants and young children not more than 5 per cent;
semi-solid formulations, 10–20 per cent;
camphor spirit, 1–10 per cent;
internal use: *Mean daily dose*: 30–300 mg.

Method of Application
Topical or for inhalation: liquid or semi-solid formulations.
Internal use: liquid or semi-solid formulations.

Medicinal Actions
External use: bronchosecretolytic, hyperaemia-inducing
Internal use: cardiovascular tonic, respiratory analeptic, bronchospasmolytic.

Carvi aetheroleum
(Caraway oil)

Banz No. 22a of 1 Feb. 1990

Official Name
Carvi aetheroleum, caraway oil

Description
Caraway oil, consisting of the volatile oil obtained from ripe fruits of *Carum carvi* L. and preparations of this in effective doses.
Caraway oil mainly contains D-carvone.

Indications
Indigestion symptoms such as mild colicky pain in gastrointestinal tract, flatulence and sensation of fullness.

Contraindications
None reported.

Side Effects
None reported.

Interactions
None reported.

Dosage
Unless otherwise prescribed,
Mean daily dose: 3–6 drops.

Method of Application
Volatile oil and galenical preparations made of it for oral administration.

Medicinal Actions
Spasmolytic, antimicrobial.

Carvi fructus
(Caraway seed)

Banz No. 22a of 1 Feb. 1990

Official Name
Carvi fructus, caraway seed

Description
Caraway seed, consisting of ripe, dried fruits of *Carum carvi* L. and preparations of this in effective doses.
Caraway seed contains volatile oil.

Indications
Loss of appetite
Indigestion symptoms such as mild colicky pain in gastrointestinal tract, flatulence and sensation of fullness.

Contraindications
None reported.

Side Effects
None reported.

Interactions
None reported.
Dosage
Unless otherwise prescribed,
1.5–6g of the drug; preparations in equivalent amounts.

Method of Application
Freshly crushed drug for infusions, also other galenical preparations for oral administration.

Medicinal Actions
Spasmolytic, antimicrobial.

Caryophylli flos
(Clove)

Banz No. 223 of 30 Nov. 1985

Official Name
Caryophylli flos, clove

Description
Clove, consisting of the hand-picked and dried flower buds of *Syzygium aromaticum* (L.) Merrill et L. M. Perry (synonyms *Jambosa caryophyllus* [Sprengel] Niedenzu; *Eugenia caryophyllata* Thunberg) and preparations of these in effective doses.
The plant drug contains not less than 14 per cent (v/w) of volatile oil, with reference to the dried drug.

Indications
Inflammatory changes in oral and pharyngeal mucosa.
In dentistry to relieve local pain.

Contraindications
None reported.

Side Effects
In concentrated form oil of cloves is irritant.

Interactions
None reported.

Dosage
Unless otherwise prescribed,
In mouth washes equivalent to 1−5 per cent of the volatile oil; in dentistry: undiluted volatile oil.

Method of Application
Powdered drug, whole or comminuted drug to obtain the volatile oil, also other galenical preparations for topical use.

Medicinal Actions
Antiseptic, antibacterial, antifungal, antiviral, local anaesthetic, spasmolytic.

Centaurii herba
(Centaury herb)

Banz No. 122 of 6 Jul. 1988

Official Name
Centaurii herba, centaury herb

Description
Centaury herb, consisting of the dried aerial parts of flowering specimens of *Centaurium minus* Moench (synonyms *Centaurium umbellatum* Gilibert, *Erythraea centaurium* [L.]

Persoon) and preparations of these in effective doses.
The bitter index of the plant drug is not less than 2,000.

Indications
Loss of appetite; indigestion.

Contraindications
None reported.

Side Effects
None reported.

Interactions
None reported.

Dosage
Unless otherwise prescribed,
Mean daily dose: 6 g of the drug; preparations in equivalent amounts. Extract (*EB* 6): daily dose 1−2 g.

Method of Application
Minced drug for infusions and other bitter preparations for oral administration.

Medicinal Actions
Increases gastric fluid production.

Coffeae carbo
(Coffee charcoal)

Banz No. 85 of 5 May 1988

Official Name
Coffeae carbo, coffee charcoal

Description
Coffee charcoal, consisting of ground outer parts of the green, dried seed of *Coffea arabica* L. s. l., *Coffea liberica* Bull. ex Hiern, *Coffea canephora* Pierre ex Froehner and other coffee species which have been roasted until blackish brown and carbonized, and also preparations of these in effective doses.

Indications
Nonspecific acute diarrhoea; topical application for mild inflammation of oral and pharyngeal mucosa.

Contraindications
None reported.

Side Effects
None reported.

Interactions
None reported.

Note
Coffee charcoal is highly adsorbent and may limit absorption of other medicinal agents given concurrently.

Dosage
Unless otherwise prescribed,
Mean daily dose 9 g; preparations in equivalent amounts.

Method of Application
Ground coffee charcoal and preparations of it for oral administration and for local applications.

Period of Application
A doctor must be consulted if the diarrhoea persists for more than 3 or 4 days.

Medicinal Actions
Adsorbent, astringent.

Colchicum autumnale
(Meadow saffron)

Banz No. 173 of 18 Sep. 1986

Official Names
Colchici semen, meadow saffron seed
Colchici tuber, meadow saffron tubers
Colchici flos, meadow saffron flowers

Description
The plant drug consists of seeds collected and dried in June/July,
or tubers collected, cut up and dried in July/August,
or fresh flowers collected in late summer and in autumn of *Colchicum autumnale* L. and preparations of these in effective doses.
Colchicum autumnale contains colchicine as the active principle; the seed contains not less than 0.4% (*DAC* 1979, stock)

Indications
Acute attacks of gout; familial Malta fever.

Contraindications
Pregnancy.
Note
Caution is indicated with elderly and weak patients and those with cardiac, renal or gastrointestinal disease.

Side Effects
None reported.

Interactions
None reported.

Dosage
Unless otherwise prescribed,
during acute attack per os, initial dose equivalent to 1 mg of colchicine, followed by 0.5−1.5 mg every 1 or 2 hours until pain subsides.
The total daily dose should not exceed 8 mg of colchicine.
To prevent attacks and treat familial Malta fever, daily oral dose equivalent to 0.5−1.5 mg of colchicine.

Method of Application
Minced drug, fresh plant extract and other galenical preparations for oral administration.

Medicinal Actions
Antichemotactic, antiinflammatory and -pyretic, antimitotic.

Condurango cortex
(Condurango [eagle vine] bark)

Banz No. 193a of 15 Oct. 1987

Official Name
Condurango cortex, condurango bark

Description
Condurango bark, consisting of the dried bark from branches and trunks of *Marsdenia condurango* Reichenbach fil. and preparations of this in effective doses.
The plant drug contains bitter principles such as condurangin.

Indications
Loss of appetite.

Contraindications
None reported.

Side Effects
None reported.

Interactions
None reported.

Dosage
Unless otherwise prescribed,
Daily dose
aqueous extract (*EB* 6): 0.2−0.5 g;
extract (*EB* 6): 0.2−0.5 g;
tincture (*EB* 6): 2−5 g; fluidextract (*Helv* VI): 2−4 g;
drug: 2−4 g.

Method of Application
Minced drug for infusions, and other bitter preparations for oral administration.

Medicinal Actions
Stimulates secretion of saliva and gastric fluid.

Crataegi folium cum flore
(Hawthorn leaves with flowers)

Banz No. 133 of 19 July 1994

Official Name
Crataegi folium cum flore; hawthorn leaves with flowers

Description
Hawthorn leaves with flowers, consisting of the dried, flowering tips of shoots of *Crataegus monogyna* Jaquind emend. Lindman or *Crataegus laevigata* (Poiret) de Candolle or other *Crataegus* species listed in the current pharmacopoeia, and preparations of these in effective doses.
The drug contains flavonoids (flavones, flavonols) including hyperoside, vitexin rhamnoside, rutin and vitexin and oligomeric procyanidines (n = 2 to n = 8 catechin and/or epicatechin units).

Phamacology, pharmacokinetics, toxicology
Actions seen with preparations of hawthorn leaves with flowers (aqueous alcoholic extracts with definitive concentration of oligomeric procyanidines and flavonoids resp.; macerations, fresh plant extracts) and individual fractions (oligomeric procyanidines, biogenic amines) in isolated organs or animal experiments were: positive inotropic action, positive dromotropic action, negative bathmotropic action, increased coronary and myocardial circulation, reduction in peripheral vascular resistance. In human pharmacological trials, with 160−900 mg given per day of aqueous alcoholic extracts (calculated for oligomeric procyanidines or flavonoids resp.) for up to 56 days the following were noted: in stage II cardiac failure (NYHA) subjective improvement and increased tolerance of effort, reduction in pressure frequency product, increase in ejection fraction, and elevation of anaerobic threshold.

Phamacokinetic studies have been limited to animal experiments, with no data available on human pharmacokinetics.

Acute toxicity studies have been done with an aqueous ethanolic dry extract (drug: extract ratio 5:1; adjusted for oligomeric procyanidines. No fatalities were seen in mice and rats given up to 3000 mg/kg BW per os or interperitoneally. Poisoning symptoms following i.p. exhibition of 3000 mg/kg BW included sedation, piloarrection, dyspnoea and tremor.

Single oral doses of the powdered drug – 3 g/kg BW for rats, and 5 g/kg BW for mice, did not prove fatal.

Rats and dogs given 30, 90 and 300 mg/kg BW of the ethanolic dry extract per os for 26 weeks showed no toxic effects. The 'no effect' dose for this extract given for 26 weeks was 300 mg/kg BW in rats and dogs. Oral doses of 300 and 600 mg/kg BW of the powdered drug given to rats for 4 weeks resulted in neither fatalities nor toxic effects.

No data are available on embryonic and fetal toxicity, fertility and postnatal development. Recent investigations of the mutagenicity of Crataegus preparations gave variable results. The mutagenic activity demonstrated for Salmonella is due to the quercetin content, and induction of SCE largely to the presence of flavone-C-glycosides, and also flavone aglycones. However, compared to the amount of quercetin taken with the food, the quercetin concentration of the drug is so low that any risk to human may be said to be practically nil.

No data are available on carcinogenicity. The data concerning genotoxicity and mutagenicity give no indication of carcinogenic risk for humans.

Indications
Reduced cardiac output corresponding to NYHA stage 2.

Contraindications
None reported.

Side effects
None reported.

Special precautions
A physician should be consulted if symptoms persist unchanged for 6 weeks or legs become oedematous. Medical advice must be sought if there is pain in the region of the heart, which may radiate to the arms, epigastrium or neck region, or in case of dyspnoea.

Use in pregnancy and during lactation
None reported.

Interactions
None reported.

Dosage
Unless otherwise prescribed, daily dose 160−900 mg of native, aqueous alcoholic extract (ethanol 45% v/v or methanol 70% v/v; drug: extract ratio 4−7:1; with defined flavonoid or procyanidine concentration) equivalent to 30−168.7 mg of oligomeric procyanidines, calculated as epicatechin, or 3.5−19.8 mg of flavonoids, calculated as hyperoside (Ger. P. 10) in 2 or 3 single doses. Crateagus fluidextract Ger. P. 10: The equivalent individual and daily dose needs to be established in clinical pharmacological studies or clinical trials.

Method of application
Liquid or solid preparations for oral use.

Period of application
Not less than 6 weeks.

Overdosage
None reported.

Special warnings
None.

Adverse effects for motorists and machine operators
None reported.

Note
The drug, aqueous, aqueous alcoholic, vinous extracts and fresh plant juice are traditionally taken to strengthen and enhance cardiovascular function.

This usage is based entirely on tradition and long-term experience.

Cucurbitae peponis semen
(Pumpkin seed)

Banz No. 223 of 30 Nov. 1985

Official Name
Cucurbitae peponis semen, pumpkin seed

Description
Pumpkin seed, consisting of ripe, dried seeds of *Cucurbita pepo* L. and cultivars of *Cucurbita pepo* L. and preparations of these in effective doses.

The seeds contain cucurbitin, free and bound phytosterols, β- and γ-tocopherol and minerals including selenium.

Indications
Irritable bladder, dysuria with benign prostatic hyperplasia stages I and II.

Contraindications
None reported.

Side Effects
None reported.

Interactions
None reported.

Dosage
Unless otherwise prescribed,
Mean daily dose: 10 g of seed; preparations in equivalent amounts.

Method of Application
Whole or coarsely chopped seeds and other galenical preparations for oral administration.

Medicinal Actions
The empirical clinical data are not supported by pharmacological trials because suitable models could not be found.

Droserae herba
(Sundew herb)

Banz No. 228 of 5 Dec. 1984

Official Name
Droserae herba, sundew herb

Description
Sundew herb, consisting of dried aerial and underground parts of *Drosera rotundifolia* L, *Drosera ramentacea* Burch ex. Harv. et Sond., *Drosera longifolia* L. p. p. and *Drosera intermedia* Hayne, and preparations of these in effective doses.
The herb contains 0.14−0.22 per cent of naphthoquinone derivatives, calculated as juglone, with reference to the anhydrous plant drug.

Indications
Spasmodic and irritable cough.

Contraindications
None reported.

Side Effects
None reported.

Interactions
None reported.

Dosage
Unless otherwise prescribed,
Mean daily dose: 3 g of the drug.

Method of Application
Liquid and solid formulations for internal and external use.

Medicinal Actions
Bronchospasmolytic, antitussive.

Echinaceae purpureae herba
(Coneflower herb)

Banz No. 43 of 2 Mar. 1989

Official Name
Echinaceae purpureae herba, coneflower herb

Description
Coneflower herb, consisting of fresh aerial parts of *Echinacea purpurea* (L.) Moench collected at flowering time, and preparations of these in effective doses.

Indications
Internal use:
Adjuvant treatment of recurrent infections in the respiratory and lower urinary tracts.
External use:
Superficial wounds with poor healing tendency.

Contraindications
External use:
None reported.
Internal use:
Progressive systemic diseases such as tuberculosis, leucopathy, collagenosis, multiple sclerosis.
Not to be given by parenteral route to patients with tendency to be allergic to daisy family, or in pregnancy.
Note
Metabolic situation of diabetics may deteriorate with parenteral applications.

Side Effects
Oral use and external applications:
None reported.
Parenteral use:
Dose-dependent rigors, short-term febrile reactions, nausea and vomiting have occurred.
Occasionally there may be an immediate allergic reaction.

Interactions
None reported.

Dosage
Unless otherwise prescribed,
Oral use:

daily dose 6–9 ml of expressed juice; preparations in equivalent amounts;
Parenteral use:
individual, depending on nature and severity of the condition and the special properties of the preparation used. Parenteral administration requires a graduated dosage scheme to be provided by the manufacturers of the particular preparation.
External use:
Semisolid formulations containing not less than 15% of the expressed juice.

Method of Application
Expressed fresh plant juice and galenical preparations of this for oral administration and for topical use.

Period of Administration
Preparations for parenteral use:
Not more than 3 weeks.
Preparations for oral administration and external use:
Not more than 6 weeks.

Medicinal Actions
In humans and/or in animal experiments, Echinacea preparations given parenterally and/or orally have shown immunobiological activity. Among other things they elevate the white cell and splenic cell count, activate the phagocytic activity of human macrophages and act as pyrogens.

Equiseti herba
(Horsetail herb)

Banz No. 173 of 18 Sep. 1986

Official Name
Equiseti herba, horsetail herb

Description
Horsetail herb, consisting of fresh or dried green, sterile shoots of *Equisetum arvense* L. and preparations of these in effective doses. The plant drug contains silica and flavonoids.

Indications
Oral use:
posttraumatic and static oedema.
Irrigation therapy for bacterial and inflammatory diseases of the lower urinary tract and for renal sand and gravel.

Contraindications
None reported.
Note
Irrigation therapy is contraindicated in patients with oedema due to reduced cardiac or renal function.

Side Effects
None reported.

Interactions
None reported.

Dosage
Unless otherwise prescribed,
internal use:
mean daily dose: 6 g of the drug, preparations in equivalent amounts;
external use:
10 g of the drug to 1 litre of water.

Method of Application
For oral administration, minced drug for infusions and other galenical preparations.
Note
Irrigation therapy:
Fluid intake must be high.
External applications:
Minced drug for decoctions and other galenical preparations,
and for local applications.

Medicinal Actions
Mildly diuretic.

Eschscholtzia californica
(Californian poppy)

Banz No. 178 of 21 Sep. 1991

Description
Californian poppy, consisting of aerial parts of *Eschscholtzia californica* Chamisso and preparations of these.

Pharmacological Properties, Pharmacokinetics, Toxicology
The plant drug contains alkaloids, the main alkaloid being cryptopine. This is reported to have a stimulant effect on the guinea pig uterus in a 1:1,000,000 dilution.

In mice, i.p. exhibition of the tincture (equivalent to 130 mg of the drug/kg body weight) was followed by a reduction in spontaneous motility and extension of pentobarbitone-induced sleep.

Exhibition of the tincture (equivalent to 1.75 mg of the drug/ml) prevents spasms in the rat jejunum due to $BaCl_2$.

Clinical Data

1 Used in combination other medicinal principles

Combinations with up to 5 constituents:

a) Californian poppy herb, valerian root, St. John's wort herb, passionflower herb, corydalis bulb.

b) Californian poppy herb, balm leaves, night-flowering cactus flowers, yohimbe bark, yellow horned-poppy herb, 2 homoeopathic preparations.

c) Californian poppy herb, valerian root, frangula bark, mallow flowers, peppermint leaves, sage leaves, cornflower flowers, balm leaves, hibiscus leaves, hop strobiles, squill, melilot herb, rosemary leaves, lavender flowers, passionflower herb, hawthorn leaves and flowers, rose petals, oat straw.

2 Indications claimed for the above

a) Reactive, agitated and masked depression, melancholia, neurasthenia, neuropathy, neurosis connected with an organ.

b) Autonomic and dystonic disorders, emotional instability, sensitivity to foehn, vasomotor dysfunction, autonomic and endocrine syndrome, constitutional instability of nervous system, vasomotor cephalgia, sensitivity to weather conditions.

c) Hypnotic and sedative tea.

Risks

Use in pregnancy and during lactation: investigations of use in pregnancy not available. In view of the pharmacology, avoid during pregnancy.

Evaluation

No reports from medical practitioners and/or hospitals and other empirical material relating to phytotherapeutic use of Californian poppy available to date.

As efficacy with the claimed indications has not been substantiated, clinical use cannot be recommended.

Eucalypti aetheroleum
(Eucalyptus oil)

Banz No. 177a of 24 Sep. 1986

Official Name

Eucalypti aetheroleum, eucalyptus oil

Description

Eucalyptus oil, obtained by rectifying the oil distilled from fresh leaves or terminal branches of various *Eucalyptus* species with high cineole content, e.g. *Eucalyptus globulus* La Billardiére, *Eucalyptus fructicetorum* F. von Mueller (syn. *Eucalyptus polybractea* R. T. Baker) and/or *Eucalyptus smithii* R. T. Baker. It contains not less than 70% (m/m) of 1,8-cineole. Preparations of the oil in effective doses.

Indications

Internal and external use: catarrhal conditions of the respiratory tract.

External use: rheumatic conditions.

Contraindications

Internal use: Inflammatory conditions in gastrointestinal region and bile ducts; serious liver disease.

External use: In infants and young children, eucalyptus preparations should not be applied in the facial region, and especially not near the nose.

Side Effects

On rare occasions, ingestion of eucalyptus preparations may cause nausea, vomiting and diarrhoea.

Interactions

Eucalyptus oil causes induction of the foreign-substance degrading enzyme system in the liver. This may weaken and/or shorten the activity of other medicinal agents.

Dosage

Unless otherwise prescribed,

Internal use: mean daily dose 0.3–0.6g of eucalyptus oil; preparations in equivalent amounts.

External use: 5–20 per cent in oily and semi-solid formulations; 5–10 per cent in aqueous and/or ethanolic formulations.

Volatile oil: massage in a few drops.

Method of Application
Volatile oil and galenical preparations of it for internal and external use.

Medicinal Actions
Secretomotoric,
expectorant
mildly spasmolytic
mild hyperaemic effect locally.

Eucalypti folium
(Eucalyptus leaves)

Banz No. 177a of 24 Sep. 1986

Official Name
Eucalypti folium, eucalyptus leaves

Description
Eucalyptus leaves, consisting of dried mature leaves from older trees of *Eucalyptus globulus* La Billardière and preparations of these in effective doses.
The plant drug contains volatile oil consisting mainly of 1,8-cineole and tannins.

Indications
Catarrhal conditions of the respiratory tract.

Contraindications
Inflammatory conditions in gastrointestinal region and bile ducts; serious liver disease.
In infants and young children, eucalyptus preparations should not be applied in the facial region, and especially not near the nose.

Side Effects
On rare occasions, ingestion of eucalyptus preparations may cause nausea, vomiting and diarrhoea.

Interactions
None reported.
Note
Eucalyptus oil causes induction of the foreign-substance degrading enzyme system in the liver. This may weaken and/or shorten the activity of other medicinal agents.

Dosage
Unless otherwise prescribed,
internal use: mean daily dose 4−6g of the drug; preparations in equivalent amounts.

Tincture (*EB* 6): daily dose 3−9g.

Method of Application
Minced drug for infusions and other galenical preparations for internal and external use.

Medicinal Actions
Secretomotoric,
expectorant
mildly spasmolytic.

Euphrasiae herba
(Eyebright)

Banz No. 162 of 29. Aug. 1992

Official Name
Euphrasia officinalis, eyebright
Euphrasiae herba, eyebright herb

Description
Eyebright, consisting of whole plants of *Euphrasia officinalis* L. p. p. collected at flowering time, and preparations of these.
Eyebright herb, consisting of fresh or dried aerial parts of *Euphrasia officinalis* L. p. p. and preparations of these.

Indications
Eyebright or eyebright herb preparations are used externally for lavage, compresses and eye baths to treat eye conditions connected with vascular disease and inflammation, blepharitis and conjunctivitis, for prevention of ophthalmic blennorrhoea or catarrh, inflamed, sticky eyes, for cough, colds, as a stomachic and for skin conditions.
Efficacy with the claimed indications has not been substantiated.

Risks
None reported.

Evaluation
As efficacy with the claimed indications has not been substantiated, clinical use cannot be recommended.

Farfarae folium
(Coltsfoot leaves)

Banz No. 138 of 27 Jul. 1990

Official Name
Farfarae folium, coltsfoot leaves

Description
Coltsfoot leaves, consisting of fresh or dried leaves of *Tussilago farfara* L. and preparations of these in effective doses.
The plant drug contains mucilage and tannins. Coltsfoot leaves also contain variable amounts of pyrrolizidine alkaloids with a 1,2-unsaturated necine structure, and their N-oxides.

Indications
Catarrhal conditions of the respiratory tract with cough and hoarseness, mild inflammatory changes in oral and pharyngeal mucosa.

Contraindications
Pregnancy, lactation.

Side Effects
None reported.

Interactions
None reported.

Dosage
Unless otherwise prescribed,
daily dose 4.5−6 g of the drug, preparations in equivalent amounts. The daily dose of coltsfoot tea (drug) and tea mixtures should not exceed 10 µg, the daily dose of extracts and fresh plant juice should not exceed 1 µg of pyrrolicidine alkaloids with 1,2-unsaturated necine structure including N oxides.

Method of Application
Minced drug for infusions and decoctions, fresh plant juice or other galenical preparations for oral administration.

Period of Application
Not more than 4 weeks.

Farfarae flos
(Coltsfoot flowers)
Farfarae herba
(Coltsfoot herb)
Farfarae radix
(Coltsfoot root)

Banz No. 138 of 27 Jul. 1990

Official Name
Farfarae flos, coltsfoot flowers
Farfarae herba, coltsfoot herb
Farfarae radix, coltsfoot root

Description
Coltsfoot flowers, consisting of fresh or dried inflorescences of *Tussilago farfara* L. and preparations of these.
Coltsfoot herb, consisting of fresh or dried aerial parts of *Tussilago farfara* L. and preparations of these.
Coltsfoot roots, consisting of fresh or dried underground parts of *Tussilago farfara* L. and preparations of these.

Indications
Coltsfoot preparations are used to treat and prevent diseases and symptoms in the region of the respiratory tract such as cough, hoarseness, bronchial catarrh, acute and chronic bronchitis, asthma, colds, influenza, inflammation and irritation of oral and pharyngeal mucosa, sore throat, tonsillitis, rickets, glandular swellings and scrofula, gastroenteritis, diarrhoea, to stimulate metabolism, to "cleanse the blood", as a diuretic and sudorific, and externally as a vulnerary.
Coltsfoot herb is an ingredient of various tonics for which different indications are stated.
Efficacy with the claimed indications has not been substantiated.

Risks
All parts of the coltsfoot plant contain variable amounts of toxic pyrrolizidine alkaloids. The health risk of using medicinal plants with toxic pyrrolizidine alkaloids is discussed elsewhere.

Evaluation
In view of the risk and as efficacy with the

claimed indications has not been substantiated, clinical use cannot be recommended.

Filipendula ulmaria
(Meadowsweet)

Banz No. 43 of 2 Mar. 1989

Official Name
Spiraeae flos, meadowsweet flowers
Spiraeae herba, meadowsweet herb

Description
Meadowsweet flowers, consisting of the dried flowers of *Filipendula ulmaria* (L.) Maximowicz (synonym *Spiraea ulmaria* L.) and preparations of these in effective doses.
Meadowsweet herb, consisting of the dried aerial parts of *Filipendula ulmaria* (L.) Maximowicz (synonym *Spiraea ulmaria* L.) collected at flowering time and preparations of these in effective doses.
The plant drug contains flavonoids, phenolglycosides (mainly in the flowers) and volatile oil.

Indications
Colds
Externally: rheumatic conditions affecting muscles and joints, blunt traumas such as contusions, strains, sprains, bruises, haematomas, etc.

Contraindications
None reported.

Note
Meadowsweet flowers contain salicylates. They should therefore not be used in cases of salicylin hypersensitivity.

Side Effects
None reported.

Interactions
None reported.

Dosage
Unless otherwise prescribed,
Daily dose 2.5–3.5g of meadowsweet flowers or 4–5g of meadowsweet herb; preparations in equivalent amounts.

Method of Application
Minced drug and other galenical preparations as infusions. 1 cup of the infusion to be taken as hot as possible several times daily.

Foeniculi fructus
(Fennel)

Banz No. 74 of 19 April 1991

Official name
Foeniculi fructus, fennel

Description
Fennel, consisting of dried, ripe fruits of *Foeniculum vulgare* Miller var. *vulgare* (Miller) Thellung, and preparations of these in effective doses. The drug contains not less than 4% of volatile oil with not more than 5% of estragon.

Uses
Dyspeptic symptoms, e.g. mild spasmodic gastrointestinal symptoms, sensation of fullness, flatus. Catarrhal upper respiratory tract conditions.
Fennel syrup, fennel honey:
Catarrhal upper respiratory tract conditions in children.

Contraindications
Dried drug for teas; preparations with volatile oil content comparable to teas. None known.
Other preparations:
Pregnancy.

Side effects
In individual cases, allergic reactions of skin and respiratory tract.

Interaction with other drugs
None reported.

Dosage
Unless otherwise prescribed, daily dose 5–7g of the drug, 10–20g of fennel syrup (EB6) or fennel honey (EB6), 5–7,5g of compound tincture of fennel (EB6), preparations in accord with this.

Method of application
Minced drug for teas, tea-type products and other galenic preparations for oral use.

Period of application
Fennel preparations should not be taken for extended periods (several weeks) unless a physician or pharmacist is consulted.

Note
Fennel syrup, fennel honey:
Diabetics must take account of the sugar content, which is . . . (as stated by manufacturer) carbohydrate units.

Actions
Encourages gastrointestinal motility, with higher concentrations spasmolytic. Experimental work has shown secretolytic actions for anethol and fenchone; aqueous fennel extracts increase mucociliary activity in frog ciliary epithelium.

Frangulae cortex
(Frangula bark)

Banz No. 133 of 21 July 1993

Official name
Frangulae cortex, frangula bark

Description
Frangula bark, consisting of dried bark from trunks and branches of *Rhamnus frangula* L. (*Frangula alnus* Miller) and preparations of this in effective doses.
The drug contains anthranoids, mainly of emodin, physcion and chrysophanol type. The drug must meet the requirements of the current pharmacopoeia.

Phamacology, pharmacokinetics, toxicology
1,8-dihydroanthacene derivatives have laxative actions. These are mainly due to an action on colon motility, inhibiting stationary and stimulating propulsive contractions. This results in accelerated passage and, due to the reduction in contact time, a reduction in fluid absorption. Stimulation of active chloride secretion also causes water and electrolytes to be secreted.

Systematic studies on the kinetics of frangula bark preparations are still outstanding, but it may be said that the aglycones are absorbed in the upper duodenum. Glycosides with β-glycosidic bonds are prodrugs and neither split nor absorbed in the upper gastrointestinal tract. They are degraded to anthrones by bacterial enzymes in the large intestine. Anthrones are the laxative metabolite.

Small quantities of active metabolites of other anthranoids such as rhein pass into mother's milk, but no laxative effect has been noted in breast-fed infants. Placental passage of rhein was found to be extremely low in animal experiments.

Drug preparations have greater general toxicity than the pure glycosides, probably because of the aglycone content. No data are available on genotoxicity of the drug or preparations of it. Aloe emodin, emodin, physcion and chrysophanol have given partly positive results. Carcinogenic properties have not been investigated.

The fresh drug contains anthrones and must therefore be stored for at least one year before it is used, or aged artificially by heating in air. Inappropriate use, e. g. of fresh drug, results in violent vomiting, sometimes with spasms.

Indications
Chronic constipation.

Contraindications
Intestinal obstruction, acute inflammatory intestinal diseases, e. g. Crohn's disease, ulerative colitis, appendicitis; abdominal pain of unknown origin. Children under 12. Pregnancy.

Side effects
In individual cases, colicky gastrointestinal symptoms. The dose needs to be reduced in that case. Chronic use/abuse: Loss of electrolytes, above all potassium, proteinuria and haematuria; pigmentation of intestinal mucosa (pseudomelanosis coli) which, however, is harmless and pigmentation of intestinal mucosa (pseudomelanosis coli) which, however, is harmless and normally disappears once the drug is discontinued, Potassium loss may cause functional cardiac disor-

ders and muscular weakness, especially if cardiac glycosides, diuretics or adrenocortical steroids are taken concurrently.

Special precautions
Stimulant laxatives should not be taken for periods of more than 1 or 2 weeks unless advised by a physician.

Use during pregnancy and lactation
Because of inadequate toxicological studies, not to be used during pregnancy and lactation.

Interactions
Chronic use/abuse may enhance the actions of cardiac glycosides and affect those of anti-arrhythmic drugs because of potassium loss. Potassium losses may be increased by combination with thiazide diuretics, adrenocortical steroids and liquorice root.

Dosage and method of application
Minced drug, powdered drug or dry extracts for infusions, decoctions, cold maceration or elixirs. Liquid or solid preparations for oral use only.
Unless otherwise prescribed,
20−30 mg of hydroxyanthracene derivatives/day, calculated as glucofrangulin A.
The correct individual dose is the lowest dose required to produce soft, formed stools.

Note
The formulation should permit daily doses that are less than usual.

Overdosage
Measures to balance electrolytes and fluids.

Specific warning
Use of stimulant laxatives for more than a short period may aggravate the constipation. The preparation should only be used if changes in diet or use of bulking agents do not give the desired results.

Motorists and machine operators
No negative effects known.

Galeopsidis herba
(Hemp-nettle herb)

Banz No. 76 of 24 Apr. 1987

Official Name
Galeopsidis herba, hemp-nettle herb

Description
Hemp-nettle herb, consisting of dried aerial parts of *Galeopsis segetum* Necker (synonym *Galeopsis ochroleuca* Lamarck) collected at flowering time and preparations of these in effective doses.
The plant drug contains tannins and saponins.

Indications
Minor catarrhal conditions of the respiratory passages.

Contraindications
None reported.

Side Effects
None reported.

Interactions
None reported.

Dosage
Unless otherwise prescribed,
Mean daily dose 6 g of the drug; preparations in equivalent amounts.

Method of Application
Minced drug for infusions and other galenical preparations for oral administration.

Gentianae radix
(Gentian root)

Banz No. 223 of 30 Nov. 1985

Official Name
Gentianae radix, gentian root

Description
Gentian root, consisting of the dried, unfermented roots and rhizomes of *Gentiana lutea* L. with a bitter index of not less than 10,000, and preparations of these in effective doses.

The plant drug contains bitter principles (amarogentin, gentiopicroside) and the bitter tasting gentiobiose.

Indications
Digestive disorders such as loss of appetite, sensation of fullness, flatulence.

Contraindications
Peptic ulcers.

Side Effects
Headaches may occasionally develop in individuals who have the disposition.

Interactions
None reported.

Dosage
Unless otherwise prescribed,
Daily dose tincture (*EB* 6) 1−3g; fluidextract (*EB* 6) 2−4g; drug 2−4g.

Method of Application
Minced drug and dry extracts for infusions, bitter formulations for oral administration.

Medicinal Actions
The main active constituents are the drug's bitter principles. These stimulate the taste receptors and hence stimulate the secretion of saliva and gastric fluid.
Gentian root is therefore considered to be not merely an amarum (purum) but in consequence also a roborant and tonic.
Animal experiments point to an increase in the volume of bronchial secretions.

Hamamelidis folium et cortex
(Witch hazel leaves and bark)

Banz No. 154 of 21 Aug. 1985

Official Name
Hamamelidis folium, witch hazel leaves
Hamamelidis cortex, witch hazel bark
Fresh leaves and branches of *Hamamelis virginiana L.*

Description
Witch hazel leaves, consisting of dried leaves of *Hamamelis virginiana* L. and preparations of these in effective doses. The plant drug contains 3−8 per cent of tannins, mainly gallotannins, flavonoids and volatile oil.

Witch hazel bark, consisting of dried bark from the stems and branches of *Hamamelis virginiana* L. and preparations of these in effective doses.

The plant drug contains not less than 4 per cent of tannins. Characteristic constituents of witch hazel bark are β-hamamelitannin and γ-hamamelitannin. The drug also contains the depside ellagtannin, catechol derivatives and free gallic acid.

Fresh leaves and branches of *Hamamelis virginiana* L., consisting of fresh leaves and branches collected in spring and early summer for the production of steam-distilled Hamamelis water.

Indications
Minor skin trauma, local inflammation of skin and mucosa;
haemorrhoids, varicose veins.

Contraindications
None reported.

Side Effects
None reported.

Interactions
None reported.

Dosage
External use
Witch hazel distilled (Hamamelis water): undiluted or diluted with water 1:3 for compresses, 20−30 per cent in semisolid formulations.
Formulations using the extract: semisolid and liquid formulations equivalent to 5−10 per cent of the drug.
Drug: decoctions of 5−10g of the drug to 1 cup (*c.* 250ml) of water for compresses and lavage/irrigation.
Internal use (mucosa):
Suppositories: 1−3 times daily amount of a formulation equivalent to 0.1−1g of the drug;
other preparations: several times daily amount of a formulation equivalent to 0.1−1g of the drug; Hamamelis water undiluted or diluted with water.

Method of Application
Witch hazel leaves and bark:
Minced drug or extracts for external and internal use.
Fresh witch hazel leaves and branches:
Steam distilled for external and internal use.

Medicinal Actions
Astringent, antiinflammatory, local styptic.

Hederae helicis folium
(Ivy leaves)

Banz No. 122 of 6 Jul. 1988

Official Name
Hederae helicis folium, ivy leaves

Description
Ivy leaves consisting of the dried leaves of *Hedera helix* L. and preparations of these in effective doses.
The plant drug contains saponins.

Indications
Catarrhal conditions of the respiratory tract; symptomatic treatment of chronic inflammatory disease of the bronchi.

Contraindications
None reported.

Side Effects
None reported.

Interactions
None reported.

Dosage
Unless otherwise prescribed,
Mean daily dose 0.3 g of the drug; preparations in equivalent amounts.

Method of Application
Minced drug and other galenical preparations for oral administration.

Medicinal Actions
Expectorant
spasmolytic
skin and mucosal irritant.

Hippocastani semen
(Horse chestnut seed)

Banz No. 71 of 15 April 1994

Official Name
Hippocastani semen, (Horse chestnut seed)/ dry extract (Ger. P. 10) of horse chestnut seed

Description
A dry extract made from horse chestnut seed (Ger. P. 10) with a triterpene glycoside concentration of 16−20% (calculated as anhydrous aescin).

Phamacology, pharmacokinetics, toxicology
The main active principle in horse chestnut seed extract, the triterpene glycose mixture aescin, has shown antiexudative and vascular sealing properties in various experimental models. There are indications that horse chestnut seed extract reduces lysosomal enzyme activity which is elevated with chronic diseases of the veins, preventing degradation of glycocalyx (mucopolysaccharides) in the region of the capillary wall. Reduced vascular permeability prevents filtration of small-molecule proteins, electrolysis and water into the interstitial spaces.

In human pharmacological studies, the drug, compared to placebo, produced significant reduction in transcapillary filtration, and in a number of randomized double-blind trials and cross-over trials gave significant improvement in symptoms of chronic venous dysfunction (feeling of tiredness, heaviness, tension, pruritus, pain and swelling of legs).

Studies to give orientation for horse chestnut seed extract toxicology are available. The LD50 of horse chestnut seed extract by mouth is 990 mg/kg BW in mice, 2150 mg/kg BW in rats, 1530 mg/kg BW in rabbits, and 130 mg/kg BW in dogs. With horse chestnut seed extract given i. v. to rats for 8 weeks, the 'no effect' dose is between 9 and 30 mg/kg BW. Chronic exhibition for 34 weeks caused gastric irritation in dogs at 80 mg/kg BW. In rats, no toxic changes were noted with 400 mg/kg BW given per os for that period.

Indications

Treatment of symptoms resulting from diseases of leg veins (chronic insufficiency), e. g. pain and sensation of heaviness in legs, nighttime leg cramps, pruritus and swelling of legs.

Note

Further, non-invasive measures prescribed by the physician, e. g. elastic bandages, supporting hose or cold water treatments must be applied.

Contraindications

None reported.

Side effects

With oral use, pruritus, nausea, gastric symptoms in individual cases.

Special precautions

None.

Use in pregnancy and during lactation

No limitations known.

Interactions

None reported.

Dosage and method of application

Daily dose 100 mg of aescin, equivalent to 250–312.5 mg of the extract in retard form twice daily.

Overdosage

None reported.

Special warnings

None.

Adverse effects for motorists and machine operators

None reported.

Hyperici herba
(St. John's wort herb)

Banz No. 228 of 5 Dec. 1984 with amendment Banz No. 43 of 2 Mar. 1989

Official Name

Hyperici herba, St. John's wort herb

Description

St. John's wort herb, consisting of plants or dried aerial parts of *Hypericum perforatum* L. collected at flowering time and preparations of these in effective doses.

Indications

Internal use: Psychovegetative disorders, depression, anxiety and/or nervous restlessness. Oily St. John's wort preparations for symptoms connected with indigestion.
External use: Oily St. John's wort preparations for treatment and follow-up treatment of sharp and blunt injuries, myalgia and 1st degree burns.

Contraindications

None reported.

Side Effects

Photosensitization is possible, especially for light-skinned individuals.

Interactions

None reported.

Dosage

Unless otherwise prescribed,
Mean daily dose for internal use 2–4 g of the drug or 0.2–1.0 mg total hypericin in other formulations.

Method of Application

Minced or powdered drug, liquid and solid formulations for oral administration. Liquid and semisolid formulations for external use. Formulations made with fatty oils for external and internal use.

Medicinal Actions

Many clinical reports refer to mild antidepressant activity of the drug and preparations made with it. Experimental studies have shown hypericin to be among the monoaminoxidase inhibitors. Oily St. John's wort preparations have antiinflammatory actions.

Lavandulae flos
(Lavender flowers)

Banz No. 228 of 5 Dec. 1984

Official Name
Lavandulae flos, lavender flowers

Description
Lavender flowers, consisting of dried flowers of *Lavandula angustifolia* Miller collected before they have fully opened and preparations of these in effective doses.

The plant drug contains not less than 1.5 per cent (v/w) of volatile oil, the main constituents being linalyl acetate, linalool, camphor, β-ocimene and 1,8-cineol. The drug also contains *c.*12 per cent of Lamiaceae tannins.

Indications
Internal use: Psychosomatic conditions such as restlessness, problems going to sleep, functional epigastric symptoms (nervous stomach, Roehmheld's gastrocardial syndrome, meteorism, intestinal problems of nervous origin).
Balneotherapy: Functional cardiovascular disorders.

Contraindications
None reported.

Side Effects
None reported.

Interactions
None reported.

Dosage
Unless otherwise prescribed,

Internal use:
As tea: 1−2 teaspoonfuls of the drug per cup
Lavender oil: 1−4 drops (*c.* 20−80 mg), e.g. on a lump of sugar
External use in baths: 20−100 g of the drug to 20 litres of water.

Method of Application
As the drug, to prepare infusions, extracts and bath additives.

Note
Combination with other sedative and/or carminative drugs may be indicated.

Medicinal Actions
Internal use: sedative, carminative.
Adequate pharmacodynamic studies on humans and animals are still outstanding, respectively they are in motion.

Ledi palustris herba
(Labrador tea herb)

Banz No. 177a of 24 Sep. 1986

Official Name
Ledi palustris herba, Labrador tea herb

Description
Labrador tea herb, consisting of the dried herb of *Ledum palustre* L. and preparations of this in effective doses.

Indications
Labrador tea is used for rheumatic conditions and whooping cough, furthermore as an emetic, diaphoretic and diuretic.
Efficacy on the above indications has not been substantiated.

Risks
There are several reports of Labrador tea poisoning, usually due to abuse, e.g. as an abortefacient.
The volatile oil taken per os causes violent irritation of the gastrointestinal tract with vomiting and diarrhoea, as well as irritation of or damage to the kidneys and lower urinary tract.
Other symptoms described are sweating, muscular and joint pain, central excitation with states of intoxication followed by paralysis.
Toxicity of Labrador tea in low doses has not been investigated.
Labrador tea is contraindicated in pregnancy.

Evaluation
As efficacy has not been substantiated and there are risks, medicinal use is not recommended.

Medicinal Actions
Skin and mucosal irritant.
Experimentally
motility inhibitor,
extends period of sleep following exhibition
of barbiturates and ethanol,
antitussive,
antiinflammatory.

Lichen islandicus
(Iceland moss)

Banz No. 43 of 2 Mar. 1989

Official Name
Lichen islandicus, Iceland moss

Description
Iceland moss (lichen), consisting of the dried
thallus of *Cetraria islandica* (L.) Acharius s.l.
and preparations of this in effective doses.
The plant drug contains mucilage and bitter
principles.

Indications
a) Irritation of oral and pharyngeal mucosa
resulting in unproductive, dry cough.
b) Loss of appetite.

Contraindications
None reported.

Side Effects
None reported.

Interactions
None reported.

Dosage
Unless otherwise prescribed,
Daily dose 4−6 g of the drug; preparations in
equivalent amounts.

Method of Application
Indications a)
Minced drug for infusions and other galenical
preparations for oral administration.
Indications b)
Minced drug ideally for cold maceration and
other bitter preparations for oral administra-
tion.

Medicinal Actions
Emollient, mildly antimicrobial.

Lini semen
(Linseed)

Banz No. 228 of 5 Dec. 1984

Official Name
Lini semen, linseed

Description
Linseed, consisting of the dried, ripe seeds of
Linum usitatissimum L. species and preparations of these in effective doses. For the indications given in this Monograph, seeds of
different cultivars of *Linum usitatissimum*
(L.) Vav. et Ell. rank as equal. The seeds
contain bulk material (hemicellulose, cellu-
lose and lignin), fatty oil, including 52-76 per
cent of linolenic acid esters, protein, linusta-
tin and linamarin respectively.

Indications
Internal use: Habitual constipation, colon
damaged by laxative abuse, irritable colon,
diverticulitis; mucilage for gastritis and enteritis.
External use: As a poultice for local inflammation.

Contraindications
Ileus of whatever genesis.

Side Effects
None reported where posology was adhered
to and above all sufficient fluids (1:10!) were
taken.

Interactions
As with all mucilaginous drugs, absorption of
medicinal agents may be negatively affected.

Dosage
Unless otherwise prescribed,
Internal use: 1 tablespoonful of whole or "accessible" (not ground) linseed 2−3 times daily, with *c.* 150 ml of fluid each time.
2 or 3 tablespoonfuls of ground or comminuted linseed to prepare linseed mucilage.
External use: 30−50 g of linseed meal in a
moist, hot poultice or compress.

Method of Application
Internal use: seed, coarsely ground seed,
"cracked" seed or so-called "accessible" seed

with cuticle and mucosal epidermis slightly squashed, linseed mucilage and other galenical preparations.
External use: as linseed meal or linseed expeller.

Medicinal Actions
Laxative action due to bulking effect triggering peristalsis due to the dilatation stimulus; demulcent to protect mucosa.

Liquiritiae radix
(Liquorice root)

Banz No. 90 of 15 May 1985

Official Name
Liquiritiae radix, liquorice root

Description
Liquorice root, consisting of unpeeled, dried roots and root runners of *Glycyrrhiza glabra* L. and preparations of these in effective doses. The root contains not less than 4 per cent of glycyrrhizinic acid and 25 per cent of water-soluble constituents.
Liquorice root consisting of peeled, dried roots and root runners of *Glycyrrhiza glabra* L. and preparations of these in effective doses. The root contains not less than 20 per cent of water-soluble constituents.
Apart from the potassium or calcium salts of glycyrrhizinic acid (= glycyrrhizin), the drug contains a number of flavonoids of the flavanone and isoflavone series. It also contains phytosterols and coumarins.

Indications
Catarrhal conditions of upper respiratory tract and peptic ulcer.

Contraindications
Cholestatic liver disease, cirrhosis of the liver, hypertension, hypokalaemia, pregnancy.

Side Effects
Extended use and relatively high doses may produce mineralocorticoid actions in form of sodium and water retention, loss of potassium with hypertension, oedema and hypokalaemia, and, in rare instances, myoglobinuria.

Interactions
Loss of potassium due to other medicinal agents, e.g. thiazides and loop diuretics may be increased. Loss of potassium increases sensitivity to digitalis glycosides.

Dosage
Unless otherwise prescribed,
Mean daily dose liquorice root *c.* 5−15 g of the drug, equivalent to 200−300 mg of glycyrrhizin.
0.5−1 g for upper respiratory catarrh;
1.5-3.0 g for peptic ulcers; preparations in equivalent amounts.

Method of Application
Drug cut up fine or powdered for infusions, decoctions, liquid and solid formulations for oral administration (Succus Liquiritiae).

Duration of Application
Unless otherwise advised by a physician, not more than 4−6 weeks.

Note
The drug may be safely used as a flavouring agent. Extended use and relatively high doses may produce mineralocorticoid actions in form of sodium and water retention, loss of potassium with hypertension, oedema and hypokalaemia, and, in rare instances, myoglobinuria. Action may be potentiated by simultaneous exhibition of thiazides and loop diuretics.

Medicinal Actions
Controlled clinical trials have shown that glycyrrhizinic acid and its aglucone accelerate the healing of gastric ulcers. Secretolytic and expectorant actions have been demonstrated in animal experiments. Concentrations of 1:2,500 to 1:5,000 were shown to have a spasmolytic effect on isolated rabbit ileum segments.

Lupuli strobulus
(Hop strobiles)

Banz No. 228 of 5 Dec. 1984

Official Name
Lupuli strobulus, hop strobiles

Description

Hop strobiles, consisting of dried inflorescences of *Humulus lupulus* L. and preparations of these in effective doses.

The plant drug contains not less than 0.35 per cent (v/w) of volatile oil.

Other constituents are alpha- and beta-bitter acids and 2-methyl-butene-3-ol.

Indications

Psychosomatic conditions such as restlessness and anxiety states, sleep disorders.

Contraindications

None reported.

Side Effects

None reported.

Interactions

None reported.

Dosage

Unless otherwise prescribed,
single dose of the drug 0.5 g.

Method of Application

Minced or powdered drug or powdered dry extract for infusions, decoctions and other preparations. Liquid and solid formulations for internal use.

Note

Combination with other sedative plant drugs may be indicated.

Medicinal Actions

Sedative, sleep-inducing.

> **Malvae flos**
> (Mallow flowers)
>
> Banz No. 43 of 2 Mar. 1989

Official Name

Malvae flos, mallow flowers

Description

Mallow flowers consisting of dried flowers of *Malva sylvestris* L. and/or *Malva sylvestris* L. ssp. *mauritiana* (L.) Ascherson et Graebner and preparations of these in effective doses.
The plant drug contains mucilage.

Indications

Irritation of oral and pharyngeal mucosa and the unproductive, dry cough connected with this.

Contraindications

None reported.

Side Effects

None reported.

Interactions

None reported.

Dosage

Unless otherwise prescribed,
Daily dose 5 g of the drug; preparations in equivalent amounts.

Method of Application

Minced drug for infusions and other galenical preparations for oral administration.

Medicinal Actions

Demulcent.

> **Malvae folium**
> (Mallow leaves)
>
> Banz No. 43 of 2 Mar. 1989

Official Name

Malvae folium, mallow leaves

Description

Mallow leaves, consisting of dried leaves of *Malva sylvestris* L. and/or *Malva neglecta* Wallroth and preparations of these in effective doses.
The plant drug contains mucilage.

Indications

Irritation of oral and pharyngeal mucosa and the unproductive, dry cough connected with this.

Contraindications

None reported.

Side Effects

None reported.

Interactions

None reported.

Dosage

Unless otherwise prescribed,
Daily dose 5 g of the drug; preparations in equivalent amounts.

Method of Application

Minced drug for infusions and other galenical preparations for oral administration.

Medicinal Actions

Demulcent.

Mate folium
(Maté leaves)

Banz No. 85 of 5 May 1988

Official Name

Mate folium, maté leaves

Description

Maté leaves, consisting of dried stems and leaf stalks of *Ilex paraguariensis* De Saint Hilaire and preparations of these in effective doses.
The plant drug contains caffeine.

Indications

Physical and mental tiredness.

Contraindications

None reported.

Side Effects

None reported.

Interactions

None reported.

Dosage

Unless otherwise prescribed,
Mean daily dose 3 g of the drug; preparations in equivalent amounts.

Method of Application

Minced drug for infusions, powdered drug for other galenical preparations for oral administration.

Medicinal Actions

Analeptic, diuretic, positive inotropic, positive chronotropic, glycogenolytic, lypolytic.

Matricariae flos
(Chamomile flowers)

Banz No. 228 of 5 Dec. 1984

Official Name

Matricariae flos, chamomile flowers

Description

Chamomile flowers consisting of fresh or dried flower heads of *Matricaria recutita* L. (syn. *Chamomilla recutita* [L.] Rauschert) and preparations of these in effective doses. The flowers contain not less than 0.4 per cent (v/w) of volatile oil. The main constituents of the oil are (-)-α-bisabolol or bisabolol oxides A and B.

Indications

External use: Skin and mucosal inflammation, bacterial skin conditions including oral cavity and parodontium.
Inflammatory conditions and irritation of respiratory tract (inhalation).
Conditions affecting anal region and genitalia (baths and irrigation).
Internal use: Gastrointestinal spasms and inflammatory diseases of the gastrointestinal tract.

Contraindications

None reported.

Side Effects

None reported.

Interactions

None reported.

Dosage

Pour hot water (*c.* 150 ml) on to 1 heaped tablespoonful of chamomile flowers (= *c.* 3 g), cover, and put through a tea strainer after 5–10 minutes.
Unless otherwise prescribed, gastrointestinal conditions are treated by taking a cup of the freshly made tea 3 or 4 times daily between meals. For inflammation of oral and pharyngeal mucosa rinse or gargle several times daily with the freshly made tea.
External use: 3–10% infusions for compresses and lavage; for baths, 50 g of the drug to

10 litres of water; semisolid formulations equivalent to 3−10% of the plant drug.

Method of Application
Liquid and solid formulations for external and internal use.

Medicinal Actions
Antiinflammatory and antipyretic, musculotropic spasmolytic, vulnerary, deodorant, antibacterial and bacterial toxin inhibitor, stimulates skin metabolism.

Melissae folium
(Balm leaves)

Banz No. 228 of 5 Dec. 1984

Official Name
Melissae folium, balm leaves

Description
Balm leaves, consisting of fresh or dried leaves of *Melissa officinalis* L. and preparations of these in effective doses. The leaves contain not less than 0.05 per cent (v/w) of volatile oil, with reference to the dried drug. Main constituents of the volatile oil are citronellal, citral a, citral b and other mono- and sesquiterpenes.
The leaves also contain Lamiaceae tannins, triterpene acids, bitter principles and flavonoids.

Indications
Functional gastrointestinal disorders, problems going to sleep of nervous origin.

Contraindications
None reported.

Side Effects
None reported.

Interactions
None reported.

Dosage
Unless otherwise prescribed,
1.5−4.5 g of the drug to a cup as an infusion several times daily as required.

Method of Application
Minced or powdered drug, fluidextract or dry extract for infusions and other galenical preparations for oral.

Note
Combination with other sedative and/or carminative plant drugs may be indicated.

Medicinal Actions
Sedative, carminative.

Menthae arvensis aetheroleum
(Mint oil)

Banz No. 177a of 24 Sep. 1986

Official Name
Menthae arvensis aetheroleum, mint oil

Description
Mint oil, consisting of the volatile oil obtained by steam distillation followed by partial dementholisation and rectification from the fresh, flowering herb of *Mentha arvensis* L. var. *piperascens* Holmes ex Christy and preparations of these in effective doses.
The oil contains not less than 3.0 and not more than 17.0% of esters calculated as menthyl acetate, not less than 42.0% of free alcohols calculated as menthol and not less than 25.0 and not more than 40.0% of ketones calculated as menthone.

Indications
Internal use:
meteorism, functional gastrointestinal and biliary disease, catarrhal conditions of the upper respiratory tract;
External use:
myalgia and neuralgiform complaints.

Contraindications
Biliary calculi,
occlusion of bile ducts, cholecystitis, serious liver damage.
Infants and young children should not have mint-oil containing preparations applied in the region of the face, especially the nose.

Side Effects
None reported.

Interactions
None reported.

Posology
Unless otherwise prescribed,
Internal use:
mean daily dose 3—8 drops,
for inhalation 3—4 drops in hot water.
External use:
a few drops applied to the skin area; 5—10%
of the volatile oil in semisolid and oily formulations, 5—10% in aqueous and ethanolic formulations, 1—5% in nasal ointments.

Method of Application
Volatile oil and galenical preparations for internal and external use.

Medicinal Actions
carminative,
cholagogue,
antibacterial,
secretolytic,
cooling.

Menthae piperitae aetheroleum
(Peppermint oil)

Banz No. 50 of 13 Mar. 1986

Official Name
Menthae piperitae aetheroleum, peppermint oil

Description
Peppermint oil, consisting of volatile oil obtained by steam distillation from freshly collected flowering shoot tips of *Mentha piperita* L. and preparations of these in effective doses.
Peppermint oil contains not less than 4.5 and not more than 10.0 per cent (w/w) of esters calculated as menthyl acetate, not less than 44.0 per cent (w/w) of free alcohols calculated as menthol and not less than 15.0 and not more than 32.0 per cent (w/w) of ketones calculated as menthone.

Indications
Internal use:
spasms in area of gastrointestinal tract and bile ducts; irritable colon; catarrhal conditions of upper respiratory tract; inflammation of oral mucosa;

External use:
Muscular and nerve pain.

Contraindications
Occlusion of bile ducts, cholecystitis, serious liver damage.
Infants and young children should not have peppermint-oil containing preparations applied in the region of the face, especially the nose.

Side Effects
None reported.

Interactions
None reported.

Posology
Unless otherwise prescribed,
Internal use:
mean daily dose 6—12 drops,
for inhalation, 3—4 drops in hot water;
for irritable colon:
average single dose 0.2 ml
mean daily dose 0.6 ml
with enteric coating.
External use:
a few drops massaged into the affected skin area; 5—10% of the volatile oil in semisolid and oily formulations, 5—10% in aqueous and ethanolic formulations, 1—5% in nasal ointments.

Method of Application
Volatile oil and galenical preparations for internal and external use.

Medicinal Actions
spasmolytic,
carminative,
cholagogue,
antibacterial,
secretolytic,
cooling.

Menthae piperitae folium
(Peppermint leaves)

Banz No. 223 of 30 Nov. 1985

Official Name
Menthae piperitae folium, peppermint leaves

Description

Peppermint leaves, consisting of fresh and dried leaves of *Mentha piperita* L. and preparations of these in effective doses.
Peppermint leaves contain not less than 1.2 per cent (v/w) of volatile oil. Other constituents are Lamiaceae tannins.

Indications

Spasms in area of gastrointestinal tract, gallbladder and bile ducts.

Contraindications

None reported.

Side Effects

None reported.

Interactions

None reported.

Posology

Unless otherwise prescribed,
Oral administration:
3–6 g of the drug, 5–15 g of the tincture (*EB* 6), preparations in equivalent amounts.

Method of Application

Minced drug for infusions, extracts of peppermint leaves for internal use.

Note

A separate monograph is available for peppermint oil.

Medicinal Actions

Direct spasmolytic effect on smooth musculature of digestive tract; choleretic and carminative.

Myrrha
(Myrrh)

Banz No. 193a of 15 Oct. 1987

Official Name

Myrrha, myrrh

Description

Myrrh, consisting of the air-dried gum resin from the stem of *Commiphora molmol* Engler and preparations of these in effective doses.
Myrrh may also derive from other *Commiphora* species, providing the chemical composition is comparable.

Indications

Topical treatment of minor inflammatory changes in oral and pharyngeal mucosa.

Contraindications

None reported.

Side Effects

None reported.

Interactions

None reported.

Posology

Unless otherwise prescribed,
Tincture of myrrh: dab on undiluted tincture 2 or 3 times daily or use 5–10 drops to a glass of water for rinsing or as a gargle.
Tooth powders containing equivalent of 10% of the powdered drug.

Method of Application

Powdered drug, tincture of myrrh and other galenical preparations for topical use.

Medicinal Actions

astringent.

Myrtilli folium
(Bilberry leaves)

Banz No. 76 of 23 Apr. 1987

Official Name

Myrtilli folium, bilberry leaves

Description

Bilberry leaves, consisting of the leaves of *Vaccinium myrtillus* L. and preparations of these in effective doses.

Indications

Bilberry leaves are used to treat diabetes mellitus and for the prevention and treatment of diseases and symptoms affected the gastrointestinal tract, kidneys and lower urinary tract, respiratory tract, rheumatic conditions, gout, skin conditions, haemorrhoidal conditions, peripheral vascular conditions, functional heart disease and to "stimulate metabolism and cleanse the blood".

Efficacy on the above indications has not been substantiated.

Risks

Relatively high dosages or extended use may cause chronic poisoning. In animal experiments this may initially take the form of cachexia, anaemia, icterus, acute states of excitation and dystonia and ultimately, with chronic exhibition of 1.5 g/kg/die, prove fatal.

Evaluation

As efficacy has not been substantiated and there is a risk involved, clinical use of bilberry leaves cannot be recommended.

Myrtilli fructus
(Bilberries)

Banz No. 76 of 23 Apr. 1987

Official Name

Myrtilli fructus, bilberries

Description

Bilberries, consisting of the dried, ripe fruits of *Vaccinium myrtillus* L. and preparations of these in effective doses.
The plant drug contains tannins, anthocyans and flavone glycosides.

Indications

Nonspecific, acute diarrhoea.
Local treatment of minor inflammatory changes in oral and pharyngeal mucosa.

Contraindications

None reported.

Side Effects

None reported.

Interactions

None reported.

Posology

Daily dose 20–60 g of the drug, for topical use as 10% decoct; preparations in equivalent amounts.

Method of Application

The dried drug for decoctions and other galenical preparations for oral administration and for topical applications.

Duration of Application

A physician should be consulted if diarrhoea persists for more than 3 or 4 days.

Medicinal Actions

astringent.

Ononidis radix
(Rest-harrow root)

Banz No. 76 of 23 Apr. 1987

Official Name

Ononidis radix, rest-harrow root

Description

Rest-harrow root, consisting of the dried roots and rhizomes of *Ononis spinosa* L. collected in autumn and preparations of these in effective doses.
The plant drug contains isoflavonoids such as ononin and small amounts of volatile oil.

Indications

Irrigation of lower urinary tract to treat inflammatory conditions; irrigation to prevent and treat renal sand or gravel.

Contraindications

None reported.

Note

Irrigation therapy is contraindicated with oedema due to reduced cardiac or renal function.

Side Effects

None reported.

Interactions

None reported.

Posology

Unless otherwise prescribed,
daily dose 6–12 g of the drug; preparations in equivalent amounts.

Method of Application

Minced drug for infusions and other galenical preparations for oral administration.

Note

Fluid intake should be high.

Medicinal Actions

Diuretic.

Origani vulgaris herba
(Marjoram herb)

Banz No. 122 of 6 Jul. 1988

Official Name
Origani vulgaris herba, marjoram herb

Description
Marjoram herb, consisting of the aerial parts of *Origanum vulgare* L. and preparations of these.

Indications
Marjoram is used to treat diseases and symptoms of the respiratory tract, cough, bronchial catarrh, as an expectorant and spasmolytic for cough, also for diseases and symptoms in the gastrointestinal region, flatulence, as a choleretic and to assist digestion, an aperitive and spasmolytic, furthermore diseases and symptoms of the urinary tract, pelvic disease, painful menstruation, as a diuretic and for rheumatic conditions, for scrofula and as a sedative and sudorific.
Marjoram herb is also contained in gargles and bath additives.
Efficacy on the above indications has not been substantiated.

Risks
None reported.

Evaluation
As efficacy has not been substantiated, clinical use cannot be recommended.

Orthosiphonis folium
(Java tea leaves)

Banz No. 50 of 13 Mar. 1986

Official Name
Orthosiphonis folium, Java tea leaves

Description
Java (or Indian kidney) tea leaves, consisting of the dried leaves and tips of *Orthosiphon spicatus* (Thunberg) Baker (Synonym *Orthosiphon stamineus* Bentham) and preparations of these in effective doses.

The plant drug contains lipophilic flavones (such as sinensetin, scutellarein tetramethylether and eupatorin), volatile oil and relatively large amounts of potassium salts.

Indications
Irrigation therapy for bacterial and inflammatory diseases of the lower urinary tract and for renal sand or gravel.

Contraindications
None reported.
Note
Irrigation therapy is contraindicated with oedema due to reduced cardiac or renal function.

Side Effects
None reported.

Interactions
None reported.

Posology
Daily dose 6–12 g of the drug; preparations in equivalent amounts.

Method of Application
Minced drug for infusions and other galenical preparations for oral administration.
Note
Fluid intake should be high.

Medicinal Actions
Diuretic
mildly spasmolytic.

Passiflorae herba
(Passion flower herb)

Banz No. 223 of 30 Nov. 1985

Official Name
Passiflorae herba, passion flower herb

Description
Passion flower herb, consisting of the fresh or dried aerial parts of *Passiflora incarnata* L. and preparations of these in effective doses.
The plant drug contains flavonoids (vitexin), maltol, coumarin derivatives and small amounts of volatile oil.
The concentration of harmala alkaloids var-

ies and must not be greater than 0.01 per cent.

Indications
Nervous restlessness.

Contraindications
None reported.

Side Effects
None reported.

Interactions
None reported.

Posology
Daily dose 4−8 g of the drug; preparations in equivalent amounts.

Method of Application
Minced drug for infusions and other galenical preparations for internal use.

Medicinal Actions
Inhibition of motility has been established in a number of animal experiments.

Piceae turiones recentes
(Young spruce or fir shoots)

Banz No. 193 of 15 Oct. 1987

Official Name
Piceae turiones recentes, young spruce or fir shoots

Description
Preparations made of fresh shoots of *Picea abies* (L.) Karsten and/or *Abies alba* Miller (Syn. *Abies pectinata* [Lamarck] de Candolle) about 10−15 cm in length collected in spring.
The shoots contain volatile oil.

Indications
Internal use: catarrhal conditions of respiratory passages.
External use: minor muscle or nerve pain.

Contraindications
None reported.

Side Effects
None reported.

Interactions
None reported.

Posology
Unless otherwise prescribed,
Internal use:
mean daily dose 5−6 g of the drug; preparations in equivalent amounts.
External use:
in baths equivalent of 200−300 g of the drug to a full bath.

Method of Application
Galenical preparations for internal and external use.

Medicinal Actions
Secretolytic, mildly antiseptic, rubefacient.

Pini aetheroleum
(Pine needle oil)

Banz No. 154 of 21 Aug. 1985

Official Name
Pini aetheroleum, pine needle oil

Description
Pine needle oil, consisting of the volatile oil obtained from fresh needles, tips of young shoots or fresh branches with needles and tips of young shoots of *Pinus sylvestris* L. *Pinus mugo* ssp. *pumilio* (Haenke) Franco, *Pinus nigra* Arnold or *Pinus pinaster* and preparations of these in effective doses.

Indications
Internal and external use
Catarrhal conditions of the upper and lower respiratory tract.
External use
Rheumatic and neuralgic pain.

Contraindications
Bronchial asthma, whooping cough.

Side Effects
May increase skin and mucosal irritation.
May increase bronchospasm.

Interactions
None reported.

Posology

For inhalation, add a few drops to hot water and inhale the vapour.

External use

Massage a few drops into the affected area; 10—50% in liquid and semisolid formulations.

Method of Application

Ethanolic solutions, ointments, gels, emulsions or oils to rub into the skin. As a bath additive and for inhalation.

Medicinal Actions

Secretolytic, rubefacient, mildly antiseptic.

Pini turiones
(Fir shoots)

Banz No. 173 of 18 Sep. 1986

Official Name

Pini turiones, fir shoots

Description

Fir shoots, consisting of fresh or dried new shoots of *Pinus sylvestris* L. 3—5 cm in length collected in spring and preparations of these in effective doses.

Pine shoots contain volatile oil and resins.

Indications

Internal use: catarrhal conditions of upper and lower respiratory tract.

External use: minor muscle and nerve pain.

Contraindications

None reported.

Side Effects

None reported.

Interactions

None reported.

Posology

Unless otherwise prescribed,

Mean daily dose 2—3 g of the drug; preparations in equivalent amounts.

Medicated rubs: liquid or semisolid formulations containing extracts equivalent to 20—50% of the drug.

Method of Application

Internal use: minced drug for infusions, as a syrup or tincture.

External use: ethanolic solutions, in oils or ointments.

Medicinal Actions

secretolytic

mildly antiseptic

rubefacient

Plantaginis lanceolatae herba
(Ribwort plantain herb)

Banz No. 223 of 30 Nov. 1985

Official Name

Plantaginis lanceolatae herba, ribwort plantain herb

Description

Ribwort plantain herb, consisting of fresh or dried aerial parts of *Plantago lanceolata* L. collected at flowering time and preparations of these in effective doses.

Ribwort plantain herb contains mucilage, iridoid glycosides such as aucubin and catalpol, and tannins.

Indications

Internal use:

Catarrhal conditions of respiratory tract; inflammatory changes in oral and pharyngeal mucosa.

External use: inflammatory skin changes.

Contraindications

None reported.

Side Effects

None reported.

Interactions

None reported.

Posology

Unless otherwise prescribed,

Mean daily dose 3—6 g of the drug; preparations in equivalent amounts.

Method of Application

Minced drug and other galenical preparations for internal and external use.

Medicinal Actions
emollient, astringent, antibacterial.

Pollen

Banz No. 11 of 17 Jan. 1991

Official Name
Pollen.

Description
Raw pollen from different flowering plants and preparations of this in effective doses.

Indications
As a roborant in states of debility, loss of appetite.

Contraindications
Pollen allergy.

Side Effects
Very occasionally gastrointestinal problems.

Interactions
None reported.

Posology
Unless otherwise prescribed,
Daily dose 30−40 g; preparations in equivalent amounts.
Micronized pollen (< 10 μm) 3−4 g; preparations in equivalent amounts.

Method of Application
Pollen and other formulations for oral administration.

Medicinal Actions
Stimulates appetite.

Polygalae radix
(Senega root)

Banz No. 50 of 13 Mar. 1986

Official Name
Polygalae radix, senega root

Description
Senega root, consisting of dried roots and root crown of *Polygala senega* L. and/or other closely related species or a mixture of *Polygala* species and preparations of these in effective doses.
The plant drug contains saponins.

Indications
Catarrhal conditions of the upper respiratory tract.

Contraindications
None reported.

Side Effects
Irritation of gastrointestinal mucosa on prolonged use.

Interactions
None reported.

Posology
Daily dose 1.5−3 g of the drug, 1.5−3 g of the fluidextract (*EB* 6), 2.5−7.5 g of the tincture (*EB* 6); preparations in equivalent amounts.

Method of Application
Minced drug for decoctions and other galenical preparations for oral administration.

Medicinal Actions
secretolytic
expectorant

Primulae flos
(Cowslip/oxlip flowers)

Banz No. 122 of 6 Jul. 1988

Official Name
Primulae flos, cowslip/oxlip (primula) flowers

Description
Cowslip/oxlip flowers, consisting of dried whole flowers, with calyx, of *Primula veris* L. and/or *Primula elatior* (L.) Hill and preparations of these in effective doses.
The sepals of the plant drug contain saponins.

Indications
Catarrhal conditions of the respiratory tract.

Contraindications
Known allergy to primulas.

Side Effects
Gastric symptoms and nausea may occasionally occur.

Interactions
None reported.

Posology
Daily dose 2—4g of the drug, 2.5—7.5g of the tincture (*EB* 6); preparations in equivalent amounts.

Method of Application
Minced drug for infusions and other galenical preparations for oral administration.

Medicinal Actions
secretolytic
expectorant

Primulae radix
(Cowslip/oxlip root)

Banz No. 122 of 6 Jul. 1988

Official Name
Primulae radix, cowslip/oxlip (primula) root

Description
Cowslip/oxlip root, consisting of dried whole rhizomes of *Primula veris* L. and/or *Primula elatior* (L.) Hill and preparations of these in effective doses. The drug contain saponins.

Indications
Catarrhal conditions of the respiratory tract.

Contraindications
None reported.

Side Effects
Gastric symptoms and nausea may occasionally occur.

Interactions
None reported.

Posology
Daily dose 0.5—1.5g of the drug, 1,5—3g of the tincture (*Austr. P.* 9); preparations in equivalent amounts.

Method of Application
Minced drug for infusions, cold maceration and other galenical preparations for oral administration.

Medicinal Actions
secretolytic
expectorant

Psyllii semen
(Psyllium (flea seed))

Banz No. 223 of 30 Nov. 1985

Official Name
Psyllii semen, psyllium (flea seed)

Description
Psyllium (flea seed), consisting of dried, ripe seeds of *Plantago psyllium* L. (synonym *Plantago afra* L.) and of *Plantago indica* L. (synonym *Plantago arenaria* Waldstein et Kitaibel) with a swelling index of not less than 10, and preparations of these in effective doses.
The plant drug contains mucilage.

Indications
Habitual constipation, irritable colon.

Contraindications
Oesophageal or gastrointestinal stenosis.

Side Effects
Very occasionally allergic reactions, specifically with powdered drug and liquid formulations.

Interactions
None reported.

Posology
Daily dose 10—30g of the drug; preparations in equivalent amounts.

Method of Application
Whole or comminuted drug, other galenical preparations for oral administration.
Note
A separate Monograph is available for flea seed (Ispaghula) husks.

Medicinal Actions
Regulates peristalsis.

Raphani sativi radix
(Radish)

Banz No. 177 of 24 Sep. 1986

Official Name
Raphani sativi radix, radish

Description
Radish, consisting of the fresh root of *Raphanus sativus* L. var. *niger* (Miller) S. Kerner and/or of *Raphanus sativus* L. ssp. *niger* (Miller) de Candolle var. *albus* de Candolle and preparations of these in effective doses.
Radish contains mustard oil glycosides and volatile oil.

Indications
Indigestion, esp. due to dyskinesia of bile ducts; catarrhal conditions of upper respiratory tract.

Contraindications
Cholelithiasis.

Side Effects
None reported.

Interactions
None reported.

Posology
Unless otherwise prescribed,
mean daily dose 500-100 ml of the expressed juice.

Method of Application
Expressed juice for oral administration.

Medicinal Actions
encourages secretion in upper gastrointestinal tract, improves motility, antimicrobial.

Rhei radix
(Rhubarb)

Banz No. 133 of 21 July 1993

Official Name
Rhei radix, rhubarb

Description
Rhubarb, consisting of dried underground parts of *Rheum palmatum* L., *Rheum officinale* Baillon or hybrids of the two species, with stem elements, small rootles and most of the bark removed, and preparations of these drugs in effective doses.
The drug contains anthranoids, mainly of rhein and physcion type.
The drug must meet the requirements of the current pharmacopoeia.

Pharmacology, pharmacokinetics, toxicology
1,8-dihydroanthracene derivatives have laxative actions. These are mainly due to an action on colon motility, inhibiting stationary and stimulating propulsive contractions. This results in accelerated passage and, due to the reduction in contact time, a reduction in fluid absorption. Stimulation of active chloride secretion also causes water and electrolytes to be secreted.
Systematic studies on the kinetics of rhubarb preparations are still outstanding, but it may be said that the aglycones of the drug are absorbed in the upper duodenum. Glycosides with β-glycosidic bonds are prodrugs and neither split nor absorbed in the upper gastrointestinal tract. They are degraded to anthrones by bacterial enzymes in the large intestine. Anthrones are the laxative metabolite.
Small quantities of active metabolites of other anthranoids such as rhein pass into mother's milk, but no laxative effect has been noted in breast-fed infants. Placental passage of rhein was found to be extremely low in animal experiments.
Drug preparations have greater general toxicity than the pure glycosides, probably because of the aglycone content. No data are available on genotoxicity of the drug or preparations of it. Aloe emodin, emodin, physcion and chrysophanol have given partly positive results. Carcinogenic properties have not been investigated.

Indications
Chronic constipation.

Contraindications

Intestinal obstruction, acute inflammatory intestinal diseases, e.g. Crohn's disease, ulterative colitis, appendicitis; abdominal pain of unknown origin. Children under 12. Pregnancy.

Side effects

In individual cases, colicky gastrointestinal symptoms. The dose needs to be reduced in that case. Chronic use/abuse: Loss of electrolytes, above all potassium, proteinuria and haematuria; pigmentation of intestinal mucosa (pseudomelanosis coli) which, however, is harmless and normally disappears once the drug is discontinued. Potassium loss may cause functional cardiac disorders and muscular weakness, especially if cardiac glycosides, diuretics or adrenocortical steroids are taken concurrently.

Special precautions

Stimulant laxatives should not be taken for periods of more than 1 or 2 weeks unless advised by a physician.

Use during pregnancy and lactation

Because of inadequate toxicological studies, not to be used during pregnancy and lactation.

Interactions

Chronic use/abuse may enhance the actions of cardiac glycosides and affect those of antiarrhythmic drugs because of potassium loss. Potassium losses may be increased by combination with thiazide diuretics, adrenocortical steroids and liquorice root.

Dosage and method of application

Minced drug, powdered drug or dry extracts for infusions, decoctions, cold maceration or elixirs. Liquid or solid formulations for oral use.
Unless otherwise prescribed,
20–30 mg of hydroxyanthracene derivatives/day, calculated as rhein.
The correct individual dose is the lowest dose required to produce soft, formed stools.

Note

The formulation should permit daily doses that are less than usual.
Tannin-rich Rheum preparations with low anthranoid concentrations may prove constipating.

Overdosage

Measures to balance electrolytes and fluids.

Specific warning

Use of stimulant laxatives for more than a short period may aggravate the constipation. The preparation should only be used if changes in diet or use of bulking agents do not give the desired results.

Motorists and machine operators

Not negative effects known.

Salicis cortex
(Willow bark)

Banz No. 228 of 5 Dec. 1984

Official Name

Salicis cortex, willow bark

Description

Willow bark, consisting of the dried bark from young vigorous 2–3 year old branches of *Salix alba* L., *Salix purpurea* L., *Salix fragilis* L. and other equivalent *Salix* species and preparations of this in effective doses.
The bark contains not less than 1 per cent of total salicin, calculated as salicin ($C_{13}H_{18}O_7$; MW 286.3) and referring to the anhydrous drug.

Indications

Febrile conditions, rheumatic conditions, headache.

Contraindications

See under Interactions.

Side Effects

See under Interactions.

Interactions

Might take the same form as with salicylates, due to the activity-determining constituents. To date, analysis of the available scientific data has given no definite indication to this effect.

Posology

Unless otherwise prescribed,

mean daily dose equivalent to 60—120 mg of total salicin.

Method of Application
Liquid and solid formulations for internal use.

Note
Combination with sudorific plant drugs may be indicated.

Medicinal Actions
Antipyretic and antiinflammatory, analgesic.

Salviae folium
(Sage leaves)

Banz No. 90 of 15 May 1985

Official Name
Salviae folium, sage leaves

Description
Sage leaves, consisting of fresh or dried leaves of *Salvia officinalis* L. and preparations of these in effective doses.
The leaves contain not less than 1.5 per cent (v/w) of volatile oil with a high thujone concentration, referring to the dried drug.
The main constituents of the volatile oil apart from thujone are cineole and camphor. The leaves also contain tannins, diterpene bitters, triterpenes, steroids, flavones and flavone glycosides.

Indications
External use
Inflammation of oral and pharyngeal mucosa.
Internal use
indigestion; increased secretion of sweat.

Contraindications
The pure volatile oil and ethanolic extracts should not be taken during pregnancy.

Side Effects
With extended use of ethanolic extracts and the pure volatile oil may cause epileptiform seizures.

Interactions
None reported.

Posology
Unless otherwise prescribed,
internal use: 1—1.5 g of the drug or 1—2 drops of the volatile oil per cup as in infusion several times daily as required;
gargle or rinse: 2.5 g of the drug or 2—3 drops of the volatile oil to 100 ml of water as an infusion, or 5 g of the ethanolic extract to 1 glass of water;
for painting: Undiluted ethanolic extract.

Method of Application
Minced drug for infusions, ethanolic extracts and distillates for gargling, rinsing and painting as well as internal use, and as fresh expressed juice.

Note
A separate Monograph is available for *Salvia triloba* (Greek sage).

Medicinal Actions
Antibacterial, fungistatic, virustatic, astringent, secretolytic and emphractic (perspiration-inhibiting).

Sambuci flos
(Elder flowers)

Banz No. 50 of 13 Mar. 1986

Official Name
Sambuci flos, elder flowers

Description
Elder flowers, consisting of the dried, sieved inflorescences of *Sambucus nigra* L. and preparations of these in effective doses.

Indications
Colds.

Contraindications
None reported.

Side Effects
None reported.

Interactions
None reported.

Posology

Unless otherwise prescribed,
mean daily dose 10—15 g of the drug; preparations in equivalent amounts.

Method of Application

Whole flowers and other galenical preparations for infusions; 1 or 2 cups of the infusion to be taken as hot as possible several times daily.

Medicinal Actions

diaphoretic; increases bronchial secretion.

Senna
(Senna)

Banz No. 228 of 5 Dec. 1984

Official Name

1) Sennae folium, senna leaves
2) Sennae fructus acutifoliae, Alexandrian or Khartoum senna fruit
3) Sennae fructus angustifoliae, Tinnevelly senna fruit

Description

1) Senna leaves, consisting of the dried leaflets of *Cassia senna* L. (*Cassia acutifolia* Del.), known as Alexandrian or Khartoum senna, or of *Cassia angustifolia* Vahl, known as Tinnevelly senna, or of a mixture of the two species and preparations of these in effective doses. The leaves contain not less than 2.5 per cent of hydroxyanthracene derivatives, calculated as sennoside B.
2) Alexandrian senna fruit, consisting of the dried fruits of *Cassia senna* L. (*Cassia acutifolia* Del.) and preparations of these in effective doses. The fruits contain not less than 3.3 per cent of hydroxyanthracene derivatives, calculated as sennoside B.
3) Tinnevelly senna fruit, consisting of the dried fruits of *Cassia angustifolia* Vahl and preparations of these in effective doses. The fruits contain not less than 2.2 per cent of hydroxyanthracene derivatives, calculated as sennoside B.
The fruits contain lower concentrations of aloe emodin derivatives than the fruit.

Indications

For all conditions where defecation should be easy, with soft stools, e.g. anal fissures, haemorrhoids and after rectal or anal surgery.
To cleanse the intestinal tract prior to X-ray examinations and before and after abdominal surgery. Chronic constipation.

Contraindications

Ileus of whatever origin; during pregnancy and lactation only under medical supervision.

Side Effects

None reported.
Chronic use/abuse results in loss of electrolytes, esp. potassium, albuminuria and haematuria; pigments deposited in intestinal mucosa (melanosis coli); damage to myenteric plexus.

Interactions

Loss of potassium with chronic use/abuse may enhance activity of cardiac glycosides.

Posology

Unless otherwise prescribed,
mean daily dose 20—60 mg of hydroxyanthracene derivatives.

Method of Application

Minced or powdered drug, powdered dry extract for infusions, decoctions and cold maceration. In liquid or solid formulations for oral administration only.

Duration of Application

Laxatives containing anthraquinones should not be taken for extended periods. Do not take for more than 8 days unless prescribed by a physician.

Medicinal Actions

The anthraquinone glycosides are reduced to aglycone emodins by colonic microbes. These are partly absorbed. Bacteria reduce them to anthranols or anthrones which have the actual medicinal action. The laxative action is due to inhibition of water and electrolyte absorption in the colon and an effect on intestinal motility.
The Monograph was revised at the end of 1994 for limited application of maximum two weeks.

> **Serpylli herba**
> (Wild thyme, mother of thyme)
>
> Banz No. 193a of 15 Oct. 1987

Official Name
Serpylli herba, wild thyme, mother of thyme

Description
Wild thyme herb, consisting of the dried aerial parts of *Thymus serpyllum* L. collected at flowering time and preparations of these in effective doses.
The plant drug contains volatile oil consisting mainly of carvacrol and/or thymol.

Indications
Upper respiratory catarrh.

Contraindications
None reported.

Side Effects
None reported.

Interactions
None reported.

Posology
Daily dose 4−6g of the drug; preparations in equivalent amounts.

Method of Application
Minced drug for infusions and other formulations for oral administration.

Medicinal Actions
antimicrobial, spasmolytic.

> **Solidago**
> (Golden rod)
>
> Banz No. 193a of 15 Oct 1987

Official Name
Solidaginis virgaureae herba, true golden rod herb
Solidaginis herba, golden rod herb

Description
True golden rod herb, consisting of the carefully dried aerial parts of *Solidago virgaurea* L. collected at flowering time and preparations of these in effective doses.

Golden rod herb, consisting of the carefully dried aerial parts of *Solidago serotina* Aiton (synonym *S. gigantea* Willdenow), *Solidago canadensis* L. and their hybrids collected at flowering time and preparations of these in effective doses.
The plant drugs contain flavonoids, saponins and phenylglycosides.

Indications
For irrigation therapy of inflammatory diseases in the lower urinary tract, for urinary calculi and renal gravel; preventative treatment of urinary calculi and renal gravel.

Contraindications
None reported.

Note
Irrigation therapy is contraindicated if there is oedema due to reduced cardiac and renal function.

Side Effects
None reported.

Interactions
None reported.

Posology
Daily dose 6−12g of the drug; preparations in equivalent amounts.

Method of Application
Minced drug for infusions and other galenical preparations for oral administration.

Note
Fluid intake should be high.

Medicinal Actions
diuretic
mildly spasmolytic
antiinflammatory and antipyretic

> **Symphyti radix**
> (Comfrey root)
>
> Banz No. 138 of 27 Jul. 1990

Official Name
Symphyti radix, comfrey root

Description

Comfrey root, consisting of fresh or dried underground parts of *Symphytum officinale* L. and preparations of these in effective doses.

The plant drug contains allantoin and mucopolysaccharides.

Comfrey root also contains varying amounts of pyrrolizidin alkaloids with 1,2-unsaturated necine structure and their N oxides.

Indications

External use

Bruises, strains, contusions, sprains.

Contraindications

None reported.

Application should be made to intact skin only; during pregnancy only under medical supervision.

Side Effects

None reported.

Interactions

None reported.

Posology

Unless otherwise prescribed,

ointments or other formulations for external use containing 5–20% of the dried drug; preparations in equivalent amounts.

The daily dose applied must not contain more than 100 µg of pyrrolizidine alkaloids with 1,2-unsaturated necine structure including their N oxides.

Method of Application

Minced drug, extracts, fresh plant juice for semisolid formulations poultices for topical application.

Duration of Application

Not more than 4–6 weeks per annum.

Medicinal Actions

antiinflammatory
promotes callus formation
antimitotic

> **Syzygii cumini cortex**
> (Jambul bark)
>
> Banz No. 76 of 23 Apr. 1987

Official Name

Syzygii cumini cortex, jambul bark

Description

Jambul bark, consisting of the dried bark from stems of *Syzygium cumini* (L.) Skeels (synonym *Syzygium jambolana* [Lam.] de Candolle) and preparations of this in effective doses.

The plant drug contains tannins.

Indications

Internal use

Nonspecific, acute diarrhoea. Topical treatment of mild inflammatory changes in oral and pharyngeal mucosa.

External use

Minor, superficial skin inflammation.

Contraindications

None reported.

Side Effects

None reported.

Interactions

None reported.

Posology

Unless otherwise prescribed,

Mean daily dose 3–6 g of the drug; preparations in equivalent amounts.

Method of Application

Minced drug for decoctions and other galenical preparations for internal and external use.

Duration of Application

A physician must be consulted if the diarrhoea persists for more than 3 or 4 days.

Medicinal Actions

Astringent.

Taraxaci radix cum herba
(Dandelion root and herb)

Banz No. 228 of 5 Dec. 1984 with
amendment Banz No. 164 of
1 Sep. 1990

Official Name
Taraxaci radix cum herba, dandelion root
and herb

Description
Dandelion root and herb, consisting of whole
plants of *Taraxacum officinale* G. H. Weber
ex Wigger s.l. and preparations of these in
effective doses.

Indications
Biliary dyskinesia; diuretic.
Loss of appetite and indigestion.

Contraindications
Occlusion of bile ducts, empyema of gall-
bladder; ileus. In cholelithiasis only under
medical supervision.

Side Effects
Gastric hyperacidity may develop, as with all
drugs containing bitter principles.

Interactions
None reported.

Posology
Unless otherwise prescribed,
infusion: 1 tablespoonful of the minced drug
to 1 cup of water;
decoction: 3−4g of the minced or powdered
drug to 1 cup of water;
tincture: 10−15 drops 3 times daily.

Method of Application
Liquid and solid formulations for oral administration.

Medicinal Actions
Choleretic and diuretic.
Aperitive.

**Terebinthinae aetheroleum
rectificatum**
(Purified turpentine oil)

Banz No. 90 of 15 May 1985

Official Name
Terebinthinae aetheroleum rectificatum,
purified turpentine oil

Description
Purified turpentine oil is the volatile oil obtained by distillation and rectification from
turpentine, an oleoresin from various species
of *Pinus*, mainly *Pinus palustris* Miller (synonym *Pinus australis* Michaux filius) and
Pinus pilaster Aiton.

Indications
External and internal use
Chronic diseases of the bronchi with marked
secretion.
External use
Rheumatic and neuralgic pain.

Contraindications
Hypersensitivity to volatile oils.
With inhalations: acute inflammation of re-
spiratory organs.

Side Effects
External use over large areas may cause toxic
symptoms incl. damage to kidneys and CNS.

Interactions
None reported.

Posology
For inhalation, add a few drops to hot water
and inhale the vapour.
External application
Massage a few drops in the affected area,
liquid and semisolid formulations containing
10−50 per cent.

Method of Application
Ointments, gels, emulsions and oils for external application; as a plaster, for inhalation
and as a bath additive.

Medicinal Actions
Rubefacient, antiseptic, reducing bronchial
secretion.

Terebinthinae Laricina
(Larch turpentine)

Banz No. 228 of 5 Dec. 1984

Official Name
Terebinthinae Laricina, larch turpentine

Description
Terebinthina laricina, Terebinthina veneta, larch turpentine, Venetian turpentine

Indications
Rheumatic and neuralgic pain, catarrhal conditions of respiratory passages, boils.

Contraindications
Hypersensitivity to volatile oils.
With inhalations: acute inflammation of respiratory organs.

Side Effects
Topical application may cause allergic skin reactions, as with all balsams.

Interactions
None reported.

Posology
External use
Liquid and semisolid formulations containing 10–20 per cent.

Method of Application
Ointments, gels, emulsions and oils for external application; as a plaster, for inhalation and as a bath additive.

Medicinal Actions
Rubefacient, antiseptic.

zygis L. or both species and preparations of these in effective doses.
The herb contains not less than 1.2 per cent (v/w) of volatile oil and not less than 0.5 per cent of phenols, calculated as thymol ($C_{10}H_{14}O$; MW 150.2) and referring to the anhydrous drug.

Indications
Symptoms of bronchitis and whooping cough.
Catarrhal conditions of upper respiratory tract.

Contraindications
None reported.

Side Effects
None reported.

Interactions
None reported.

Posology
Unless otherwise prescribed,
1–2 g of the drug to a cup as infusion, several times daily as required; fluidextract 1–2 g.
For compresses, a 5 per cent infusion.

Method of Application
Minced or powdered drug, fluidextract or dry extract for infusions and other galenical preparations. Liquid and solid formulations for internal and external use.

Note
Combination with other expectorant plant drugs may be indicated.

Medicinal Actions
Bronchospasmolytic, expectorant, antibacterial.

Thymi herba
(Thyme herb)

Banz No. 228 of 5 Dec 1984

Official Name
Thymi herba, thyme herb

Description
Thyme herb, consisting of stripped-off and dried leaves of *Thymus vulgaris* L., *Thymus*

Tiliae flos
(Lime flowers)

Banz No. 164 of 1 Sep. 1990

Official Name
Tiliae flos, lime flowers

Description
Lime flowers, consisting of the dried inflorescences of *Tilia cordata* Miller and/or *Tilia*

platyphyllos Scopoli and preparations of these in effective doses.

Indications
Colds and coughs connected with these.

Contraindications
None reported.

Side Effects
None reported.

Interactions
None reported.

Posology
Unless otherwise prescribed,
daily dose 2−4g of the drug; preparations in equivalent amounts.

Method of Application
Minced drug for infusions and other galenical preparations for oral administration.

Medicinal Actions
diaphoretic.

Tiliae folium
(Lime leaves)
Banz No. 164 of 1 Sep. 1990

Official Name
Tiliae folium, lime leaves

Description
Lime leaves, consisting of leaves of *Tilia cordata* Miller and/or *Tilia platyphyllos* Scopoli and preparations of these in effective doses.

Indications
Preparations made from lime leaves are used as a diaphoretic.
Efficacy on the above indications has not been substantiated.

Risks
None reported.

Evaluation
As efficacy has not been substantiated, clinical use cannot be recommended.

Reasons
Lime leaves are only used in a small number of phytomedicines. Proof of efficacy is not available.
Use as a filler in tea mixtures is judged safe.

Tormentillae rhizoma
(Tormentil rhizome)
Banz No. 85 of 5 May 1988

Official Name
Tormentillae rhizoma, tormentil rhizome

Description
Tormentil rhizome, consisting of the dried rhizome of *Potentilla erecta* (L.) Raeuschel (synonym *Potentilla tormentilla* Necker), with roots removed, and preparations of these in effective doses.
The plant drug contains a high concentration of tannins.

Indications
Nonspecific, acute diarrhoea; minor inflammatory changes in oral and pharyngeal mucosa.

Contraindications
None reported.

Side Effects
Sensitive patients may develop gastric symptoms.

Interactions
None reported.

Posology
Daily dose 4−6g of the drug; preparations in equivalent amounts.
Tormentilla tincture: 10−20 drops to 1 glass of water several times daily to rinse oral and pharyngeal mucosa.

Method of Application
Minced drug for decoctions and infusions and other galenical preparations for oral administration and topical use.

Duration of Application
A physician must be consulted if diarrhoea persists for more than 3 or 4 days.

Medicinal Actions
astringent

Usnea species
(Lichens)

Banz No. 80 of 27 Apr. 1989

Official Name
Usnea species, lichens

Description
Lichens, consisting of the dried thalluses of *Usnea* species, esp. *Usnea barbata* (L.) Wiggers emend. Mot., *Usnea florida* (L.) Fries, *Usnea hirta* (L.) Hoffmann and *Usnea plicata* (L.) Fries and preparations of these in effective doses.

Indications
Minor inflammatory changes in oral and pharyngeal mucosa.

Contraindications
None reported.

Side Effects
None reported.

Interactions
None reported.

Posology
Unless otherwise prescribed,
Sucking tablets containing formulations equivalent to 100 mg of the drug; 3−6 times daily 1 lozenge.

Method of Application
Formulations for sucking tablets and comparable solid formulations.

Medicinal Actions
Antimicrobial.

Uvae ursi folium
(Bearberry leaves)

Banz No. 109 of 15 June 1994

Official Name
Uvae ursi folium, bearberry leaves

Description
Bearberry leaves, consisting of dried foliage leaves of *Arcostaphylos uva ursi* (L.) Sprengel, and preparations of these in effective doses.
The dried leaves contain not less than 6.0% of hydroquinone derivatives, calculated as anhydrous arbutin, with reference to the anhydrous drug.

Phamacology, pharmacokinetics, toxicology
In vitro, bearberry leaf preparations have antibacterial actions against Proteus vulgaris, E. coli, Ureaplasma urealyticum, Mycoplasma hominis, Staphylococcus aureus, Pseudomonas aeruginosa, Klebsiella pneumoniae, Enterococcus faecalis, Steptococcus strains and Candida albicans. The antimicrobial action is thought to relate to the aglycone hydroquinone which is released from arbutin (transport form) or arbutin elimination products in alkaline urine.
A methanolic extract of the drug (50%) is reported to inhibit tyrosine activity. The extract is also stated to inhibit production of melanin from DOPA with the aid of tyrosinase and from DOPA-CHROM by autoxidation.
There are indications that following ingestion of bearberry tea (3 g/150 ml), the urine contains mainly hydroquinone glucuronide and small quantitites of hydroquinone.

Indications
Inflammatory changes in urianry tract.

Contraindications
Pregnancy, lactation. Children under 12.

Side effects
Nausea and vomiting may occur in individuals with sensitive stomachs.

Special precautions
None known.

Use in pregnancy and during lactation
Not used during pregnancy. Transfer of arbutin/hydroquinone into mother's milk has not been investigated. The drug should therefore not be used during lactation.

Interactions
Bearberry leaf preparations should not be given concurrently with medicines that cause the urine to be acid, as this reduces the antibacterial activity.

Dosage
Unless otherwise prescribed,
single dose: 3 g of the drug to 150 ml of water as an infusion or cold maceration, or 100−210 mg of hydroquinone derivatives, calculated as anhydrous arbutin.
Daily dose: up to 4 times daily 3 g of the drug, or 400−840 mg of hydroquinone derivatives, calculated as anhydrous arbutin.

Method of application
Minced drug, powdered drug for infusions or cold maceration, extracts and solid preparations for oral use.

Period of application
Drugs containing arbutin should not be taken for more than 1 week at a time and not more than 5 times a year.

Overdosage
None reported.

Special warnings
Not known.

Adverse effects for motorists and machine operators
None reported.

Uzarae radix
(Uzara root)

Banz No. 164 of 1 Sep. 1990

Official Name
Uzarae radix, uzara root

Description
Uzara root, consisting of the dried underground parts of 2−3 year old plants of *Xysmalobium undulatum* (L.) R. Brown and preparations of these in effective doses.
The plant drug contains glycosides with cardenolide structure.

Indications
Nonspecific, acute diarrhoea.

Contraindications
Treatment with cardiac glycosides.

Side Effects
None reported.

Interactions
None reported.

Posology
Unless otherwise prescribed,
adults: single initial dose 1 g of the drug or equivalent of 75 mg of total glycosides; daily dose equivalent to 45−90 mg of total glycosides, calculated as uzarin.

Method of Application
Extracts made with ethanol/water mixtures or dry extracts, made with methanol/water mixtures, for oral administration.

Duration of Application
A physician must be consulted if diarrhoea persists for more than 3 or 4 days.

Medicinal Actions
motility inhibitor; in large doses digitalis-type action on the heart.

Valerianae radix
(Valerian root)

Banz No. 90 of 15 May 1985

Official Name
Valerianae radix, valerian root

Description
Valerian root, consisting of the underground parts of *Valeriana officinalis* L.s.l., fresh or dried carefully below 40 °C, and preparations of these in effective doses.

Indications
Restlessness, problems going to sleep of nervous origin.

Contraindications
None reported.

Side Effects
None reported.

Interactions
None reported.

Posology
Unless otherwise prescribed,
infusion: 2−3 g per cup, 1 or several times daily;

tincture: ½−1 teaspoonful (1−3ml) 1 or several times daily;
extracts: equivalent to 2−3g of the drug 1 or several times daily;
external use
100g of the drug to a full bath; preparations in equivalent amounts.

Method of Application
Internal use: as expressed juice, tincture, extracts and other galenical preparations.
External use: as bath additive.

Medicinal Actions
Sedative, facilitates going to sleep.

Verbasci flos
(Mullein flowers)

Banz of 22a of 1 Feb. 1990

Official Name
Verbasci flos, mullein flowers

Description
Mullein flowers, consisting of the dried corollas of *Verbascum densiflorum* Bertolini and/or *Verbascum phlomoides* L. and preparations of these in effective doses.

Indications
Catarrhal conditions of the respiratory tract.

Contraindications
None reported.

Side Effects
None reported.

Interactions
None reported.

Posology
Unless otherwise prescribed,
Daily dose 3−4g of the drug; preparations in equivalent amounts.

Method of Application
Minced drug for infusions and other galenical preparations for oral administration.

Medicinal Actions
Emollient
expectorant

Violae tricoloris herba
(Heartsease herb)

Banz No. 50 of 13 Mar. 1986

Official Name
Violae tricoloris herba, heartsease herb

Description
Heartsease herb, consisting of the dried aerial parts of *Viola tricolor* L., mainly the subspecies *vulgaris* (Koch) Oborny and *arvensis* (Murray) Gaudin, collected at flowering time, and preparations of these in effective doses.
The plant drug contains flavonoids.

Indications
External use
mild, seborrhoeic skin conditions; milk crust of infants.

Contraindications
None reported.

Side Effects
None reported.

Interactions
None reported.

Posology
Unless otherwise prescribed,
1.5g of the drug to 1 cup of water as infusion, 3 times daily; preparations in equivalent amounts.

Method of Application
Minced drug for infusions or decoctions and other galenical preparations for topical use.

Zingiberis rhizoma
(Ginger root)

Banz No. 85 of 5 May 1988 and
Banz No. 50 of 13 Mar. 1990 and
Banz No. 164 of 1 Sep. 1990

Official Name
Zingiberis rhizoma, ginger root

Description
Ginger root, consisting of finger-lengths of peeled fresh or dried rhizome of *Zingiber officinalis* Roscoe and preparations of these in effective doses.

Indications
Indigestion; prevention of travel sickness symptoms.

Contraindications
Cholelithiasis, unless under medical supervision.

Note:
Contraindicated for hyperemesis gravidarum.

Side Effects
None reported.

Interactions
None reported.

Posology
Daily dose 2−4 g of the drug; preparations in equivalent amounts.

Method of Application
Minced drug and dry extracts for infusions; other galenical preparations for oral administration.

Medicinal Actions
Antiemetic, positive inotropic, promotes secretion of saliva and gastric fluid, cholagogue; in animals spasmolytic; in humans increased intestinal tone and peristalsis.

Chapter 6
ESCOP Monographs
**(Proposals for European Monographs
on the medicinal use of phytomedicines)**

6.1 Introduction to the Monographs

The European Scientific Cooperative on Phytotherapy (ESCOP) has been established in Cologne, Germany, in 1989 to develop uniform criteria for the evaluation of phytomedicines within the European Community. Currently 15 European scientific societies working on phytotherapy are members of ESCOP.

A European Scientific Committee has been working to establish ESCOP Monographs. Prior to publication their proposals are considered, improved and/or supplemented by the ESCOP Board of Supervising Editors, which is also international. The ESCOP Monographs are then submitted for recognition as Euro-SPCs to the Committee of Proprietary Medicinal Products (CPMP) at the European Communities Commission.

The Monographs given below have ESCOP approval*. Another 20 Monographs are under review or have been passed by the ESCOP Scientific Committee. The author of this book is a member of the Board of Supervising Editors.

---

* Original English text reprinted with kind permission of European Scientific Cooperative on Phytotherapy (ESCOP). The references to published literature used in support of a monograph at the end of the respective monographs are omitted. For monographs including references please contact: ESCOP Secretariat, Uitwaardenstraat 13, NL-8081 HJ Elburg, The Netherlands.

6.2 Alphabetical List of ESCOP Monographs (International Latin terms)

Allii sativi bulbus
Calendulae flos /
Calendulae flos cum herba
Crataegus
Frangulae cortex
Lupuli strobulus
Matricariae flos
Menthae piperitae aetheroleum
Passiflorae herba

Plantaginis ovatae semen
Sennae folium
Sennae fructus acutifoliae /
Sennae fructus angustifoliae
Taraxaci folium
Taraxaci radix
Uvae ursi folium
Valerianae radix

6.3 Approved ESCOP Monographs, in alphabetical sequence

Allii sativi bulbus
(Garlic Bulb)

(c) ESCOP – March 1992

Definition

Garlic bulb consists of the air-dried (so-called "fresh") or fully dried bulbs of *Allium sativum* L.

The material complies with the British Herbal Pharmacopoeia.

Constituents

Carefully dried, powdered material contains about 1 per cent alliin [(+)-S-allyl-L-cysteine sulphoxide) as the main sulphur-containing amino acid. Other characteristic, genuine constituents are (+)-S-methyl-L-cysteine sulphoxide, γ-glutamyl peptides, ubiquitous amino acids, steroids and adenosine.

In the presence of the enzyme alliinase, alliin will be converted to allicin (0.45 mg of allicin is considered to be equivalent to 1 mg of alliin). In turn, allicin is the precursor of various transformation products, including ajoenes, vinyldithiines, oligo- and polysulphides, depending on the conditions applied.

Material derived from garlic by steam distillation or extraction in an oily medium contains various allicin transformation products.

Action

Hypolipidaemic (cholesterol and triglyceride lowering), hypotensive, lowers blood viscosity, activates fibrinolysis, improves microcirculation, inhibits platelet aggregation, antimicrobial.

Pharmacological properties

The effects are primarily due to allicin and its transformation products.

Pre-clinical studies:

Garlic powder as well as fresh garlic and oil preparations reduced experimentally induced hyperlipidaemia and atherosclerosis.

Anti-aggregatory, antibacterial, antimycotic, antiviral, antihepatotoxic and tumor growth inhibiting actions have been shown in vitro and in vivo.

Clinical studies:

In a single dose oral administration a standardized garlic powder has been shown to lower haematocrit and plasma viscosity and to increase fibrinolytic activity and capillary blood flow in healthy volunteers. In a 30-day, double-blind investigation, a significant reduction of spontaneous platelet aggregation was shown in patients with constantly elevated spontaneous platelet aggregation using a standardized garlic powder preparation.

In double-blind studies over a period of 50 to 100 days the following significant effects have been shown with standardized garlic powder preparations and with non-standardized garlic oil extracts:

– a lowering of blood lipids (cholesterol and triglycerides) in patients with hyperlipidaemia
– a lowering of blood pressure in hypertensive patients
– an improvement of the pain-free walking distance in patients with intermittent claudication.

In a controlled study over a period of 3 years, in patients who had suffered myocardial infarction, a significant reduction of the reinfarction rate and mortality was shown using a non-standardized garlic oil extract.

Indications

Prophylaxis of atherosclerosis. Treatment of elevated blood lipid levels insufficiently influenced by diet.

Improvement of blood flow in arterial vascular disease.

Traditionally used for the relief of coughs, colds, catarrh and rhinitis.

Contra-indications
Non known.

Side effects
Alteration in the odour of skin and breath may occur.
In rare cases gastro-intestinal irritation or allergic reactions.

Use during pregnancy and lactation
No adverse effects reported.

Special warnings
None required.

Interactions
None reported.

Dosage
The equivalent of 4−10 mg of alliin (approx. 2−5 mg of allicin) daily as garlic powder or other preparations.

Mode of administration
Oral, as solid dosage forms.

Duration of administration
Not restricted. Long term treatment is generally advised in prevention of atherosclerosis and prophylaxis or treatment of arterial vascular diseases.

Overdose
No toxic effects reported.

Effects on ability to drive and use machines
Nothing reported.

References
See ESCOP Monograph Proposals, Vol. 2 (March 1992)

Calendulae flos
(Marigold Flower), and
Calendulae flos cum herba
(Marigold Flowering Herb)

(c) ESCOP – March 1992

Definition
Marigold flower consists of the dried ligulate florets (complying with the German "Standardzulassungen" or of the dried composite flowers (complying with the French pharmacopoeia and the – now invalid – AB7-DDR) of *Calendula officinalis* L.
The variety with relatively more ligulate florets ("filled" flowers) is usually used.
Fresh material may also be used, provided that when dried it complies with one of the above specifications.
Marigold flowering herb consists of the dried aerial parts of *Calendula officinalis* L., collected when in flower.
Fresh material may also be used.

Constituents
Triterpenoids (oleanolic acid glycosides and triterpene alcohols), sesquiterpenoids, carotenoids, flavonoids, polysaccharides.

Action
Wound healing, anti-inflammatory, immunomodulating.

Pharmacological properties
– Granulation stimulation – wound care in humans and in wounded rats.
– Phagocytosis stimulation in vitro, in the carbon clearance test with mice, in wounded rats and towards *Escherichia coli* in mice.
– Anti-inflammatory activity in rats and with the carrageen test in mice.
– Healing or suppression of gastric and duodenal ulcers in rats.
– Anti-tumoral activity in vivo in mice and in vitro; anti-hyperlipaemic activity (especially of the herb) in rats; choleretic activity in dogs; antibacterial, antifungal, antiviral, and antiparasitic (trichomonacidal) activity – all in vitro.

Indications

Skin and mucous membrane inflammations, badly healing wounds, mild burns, decubitus and sunburn.

Traditional uses of Calendula preparations are:

Internally for the treatment of skin infections and of *Herpes zoster* infections.

As a cholagogue and for peripheral vasodilatation.

Contra-indications

None known.

Side effects

No adverse effects confirmed.

Use during pregnancy and lactation

No adverse effects reported.

Special warnings

Non required.

Interactions

None reported.

Dosage and mode of administration

External use:

- Infusion for compresses and wound dabbing: 1–2 g/150 ml.
- Tincture for external use: either the tincture 1:10 from flowers or a tincture 1:20–1:30 from flowering herb. For wound dabbing they are applied undiluted, for compresses usually diluted 1:3 with freshly boiled water.
- Ointments.
- Freshly prepared poultice.

Internal use:

- Tea for internal use: 5 g in 100 ml water as infusion.
- Tincture for internal use.

Marigold flower and flowering herb are treated together as in traditional phytotherapy both crude drugs are used for the indications mentioned. Pharmacological data and quantitative phytochemical data delineating differences and similarities are regrettably unavailable in the literature; however, the oleanolic acid glycosides, probably important active constituents, are found in all parts of the plant.

Dosage: A cup of the tea or 5–40 drops of the tincture, 3 times a day.

Duration of administration

No adverse effects from long term use are known.

Overdose

No toxic effects reported.

Effects on ability to drive and use machines

Nothing reported.

References:

See ESCOP Monograph Proposals, Vol. 3 (March 1992).

Crataegus
(Hawthorn)

(c) ESCOP – March 1992

Definitions

Hawthorn consists of the dried flowering tops, flowers, leaves or fruits of the following *Crataegus* species.

Hawthorn flowering tops and flowers are derived from *Crataegus monogyna* Jacquin emend. Lindman or *Crataegus laevigata* (Poiret) de Candolle (*Crataegus oxyacantha* L.p.p.) or less frequently from other European *Crataegus* species, such as *Crataegus pentagyna* Waldstein et Kitaibel ex Willdenow, *Crataegus nigra* Waldstein et Kitaibel or *Crataegus azarolus* L. They contain a minimum of 0.7 per cent total flavonoids.

Hawthorn flowering tops comply with the French or German or Swiss pharmacopoeias. Hawthorn flowers comply with Pharmacopée Française or with the Deutscher Arzneimittel-Codex.

Hawthorn leaves comply, except for the presence of flowers, with the requirements of the respective pharmacopoeial monographs for Hawthorn flowering tops.

Hawthorn fruits are derived form *Crataegus laevigata* (Poiret) de Candolle or *Crataegus monogyna* Jacquin emend. Lindman and their hybrids.

The material complies with the Deutscher Arzneimittel-Codex (DAC).

Fresh materials may also be used provided that when dried they comply with their respective pharmacopoeial monographs.

Constituents

Flavonoids such as hyperoside, vitexin and vitexin-2"-rhamnoside; oligomeric procyanidins, (−)-epicatechin.

These are considered to be the main active constituents.

Action

Improves cardiac function.

Pharmacological properties

In vitro or animal experiments:

Enhances coronary blood flow and myocardial perfusion. Improves cardiac muscle contractility with an increase in the maximum pressure rise velocity of the left ventricle. Increases cardiac performance and output and lowers the peripheral vascular resistance as a parameter of the afterload; the blood pressure remains unchanged or is reduced.

Has antiarrhythmic effects; positive chronotropic as well as negative chronotropic activities have been described.

Increases the myocardium's tolerance to oxygen deficiency under hypoxic conditions.

Reduces the extent of the necrotic area in experimental myocardial infarction and stimulates revascularization after the myocardial ischaemia.

One of the mechanisms of action seems to be an inhibition of cAMP-phosphodiesterase activity.

Shows mild sedative effects at very high dose levels; cardiovascular effects can be demonstrated at significantly lower dosage.

Clinical studies:

Clinical results demonstrate an increase in cardiac performance and output, a decrease in peripheral vascular resistance, a decrease in pulmonary arterial and capillary pressure, a reduction in the pressure rate product at rest and during exercise, a rise in ergometric tolerance and an improvement in metabolic parameters.

Indications

Declining cardiac performance equivalent to stages I and II of the NYHA (New York Heart Association) classification. Cases of senile heart where digitalis is not yet required.

Sensations of pressure or constriction in the cardiac area; mild, stable forms of angina pectoris stage I NYHA.

Mild forms of dysrhythmia.

The flowering tops are traditionally used in the symptomatic treatment of nervous states, especially in cases of mild sleep disturbances.

Contra-indications

None known.

Side effects

No adverse effects reported.

Use during pregnancy and lactation

No adverse effects reported.

Special warnings

None required.

Interactions

None reported.

Dosage

Oral daily dose:

As infusions an average of 1 g of drug 3−4 times/day. Other preparations, containing a minimum of 5 mg flavonoids, calculated as hyperoside, or 10 mg total flavonoids (determined as total phenols, calculated as hyperoside) or 5 mg oligomeric procyanidins [calculated as epicatechin].

Parenteral dose:

At least 50 per cent of the oral dose.

Mode of administration

Oral, in liquid or solid dosage forms.
Parenteral, as i. m. or i. v. injections.

Duration of administration

No restriction.

Overdose

No toxic effects reported.

Effects on ability to drive and use machines

None.

References:
See ESCOP Monograph Proposals, Vol. 2 (March 1992)

Frangulae cortex
(Frangula Bark)

(c) ESCOP – October 1990

Definition
Frangula bark consists of the dried bark of the stems and branches of *Rhamnus frangula* L. [*Frangula alnus* Miller]. It contains not less than 6.0 per cent of hydroxyanthracene derivatives, calculated as glucofrangulin A (M_r 578.5).
The material complies with the European Pharmacopoeia.

Constituents
The main active constituents of the dried bark are the glucofrangulins A and B (emodin diglycosides) and the frangulins A and B (emodin mono glycosides), together with small amounts of other anthraquinone glycosides, dianthrones and aglycones.
In the fresh bark the anthrone form of the glucofrangulins, which is associated with more side effects, predominates. Therefore, before use the drug should be stored for at least 1 year or heated for $1-2$ hours at $100\,°C$ in order to oxidize the anthrones into the anthraquinones.

Action
Laxative.

Pharmacological properties
The 1,8-dihydroxyanthraquinones have a laxative action affecting mainly the colon. Fluid secretion is induced and peristalsis stimulated.

Indications
Constipation and all cases in which easy defecation with soft faeces is desirable, e. g. in cases of anal fissures, haemorrhoids and after rectal and abdominal surgery, as well as for bowel clearance before surgery and in diagnostic investigations.

Contra-indications
Inflammatory colon diseases (e. g. ulcerative colitis, Crohn's disease), ileus, appendicitis, abdominal pain of unknown origin.

Side effects
If used correctly, side effects will be minimal.
– Abdominal spasms
– Yellow or red-brown (pH-dependent) discoloration of urine by metabolites, which is harmless.
– Chronic use may cause pigmentation of the colon (pseudomelanosis coli), which is harmless and reversible after drug discontinuation.

Use during pregnancy and lactation
No data available to assess safety or risks. Not recommended during pregnancy and lactation.

Special warnings
Long term use of laxatives should be avoided. Abuse, with consequent fluid and electrolyte losses, may cause
– dependence with possible need for increased dosages
– disturbance of the water and electrolyte balance (mainly hypokalemia)
– an atonic colon with impaired function

Interactions
Hypokalemia (resulting from long term laxative abuse) potentiates the action of cardiac glycosides and interacts with antiarrhythmic drugs, with drugs which induce reversion to sinus rhythm (e. g. quinidine) and with other drugs which induce hypokalemia (e. g. corticoids, diuretics).

Dosage
Adult daily dose: drug equivalent to $20-200\,mg$ of hydroxyanthracene derivatives calculated as glucofrangulin A.
Children from 6 to 12 years: half of the adult dosage.

Mode of administration
For oral administration only, in liquid or solid dosage forms.

Duration of administration
Should not be taken for long periods.

Overdose
The major symptoms are griping and severe diarrhoea with consequent losses of fluid and electrolyte, which should be replaced.

Effects on ability to drive and use machines
None.

References
See ESCOP Monograph Proposals, Vol. 1 (October 1990)

Lupuli strobulus
(Hops)

(c) ESCOP – March 1992

Definition
Hops consists of the dried inflorescences of *Humulus lupulus* L. collected from the female plant. It contains not less than 0.3 per cent (V/m) of essential oil.
The material complies with the Pharmacopée Française.
Fresh material may also be used provided that when dried it complies with the Pharmacopée Française.

Constituents
Bitter principles (15–25%) consisting of a hard resin and a series of α-acids, principally humulone and related compounds, and β-acids, mainly lupulone and similar compounds. Volatile oil containing mainly myrcene, humulene and caryophyllene with a trace of 2-methyl-3-buten-2-ol, which will increase in amount to a maximum (approx. 0.15%) after storage of Hops for 2 years due to degradation of the humulones and lupulones. Other constituents include the chalcone xanthohumol, flavonoids and tannins.

Action
Sedative, spasmolytic, digestive stimulant.

Pharmacological properties
The sedative effect of Hops is undisputed in empirical medicine but early experiments to demonstrate this action in animals produced conflicting results. Subsequently, 2-methyl-3-buten-2-ol, given intraperitoneally to mice at high dosage levels, showed central nervous depressant activity.
Although present only in small amounts in the drug, higher levels of 2-methyl-3-buten-2-ol may be generated in vivo by metabolization of humulones and lupulones.
The effectiveness of this constituent is comparable, in the same dosage range, to that of the structurally related drug methylpentynol. Alcoholic extracts of Hops have shown a strong spasmolytic effect on isolated muscle. The stimulating effect of Hops on gastric secretion has been demonstrated in animals. Reports of oestrogenic activity in Hops have been inconclusive.

Indications
Nervous tension, excitability, restlessness and sleep disturbances and lack of appetite.

Contra-indications
None known.

Side effects
None known.

Use during pregnancy and lactation
No adverse effects reported.

Special warnings
None required.

Interactions
None reported.

Dosage
Ca. 0.5 g of the drug as an infusion or 1 to 2 ml of the tincture (1:5), once or several times daily; other equivalent preparations.

Mode of administration
Oral, as liquid or solid dosage forms.
Externally, as a bath additive.

Duration of administration
No restriction.

Overdose
No toxic effects reported; neither dependence nor withdrawal symptoms are reported.

Effects on ability to drive and use machines
Nothing reported.

References
See ESCOP Monograph Proposals, Vol. 2
(March 1992)

Matricariae flos
(Matricaria Flower)

(c) ESCOP – October 1990

Definition
Matricaria flower consists of the dried flow-er-heads of *Matricaria recutita* L. [*Chamomilla recutita* (L.) Rauschert]. It con-tains not less than 0.4 per cent V/m of blue essential oil.
The material complies with the European Pharmacopoeia.
Fresh material may also be used provided that when dried it complies with the Euro-pean Pharmacopoeia.

Constituents
Essential oil of Matricaria flower consisting mainly of $(-)$-α-bisabolol or the bisabolol oxides A and B and matricine, which is con-verted to chamazulene on distillation. Other constituents of the flower-heads include ene-yne-bicycloethers and flavone derviatives such as apigenin-7-glucoside.
These are considered to be the main active constituents.

Action
Anti-inflammatory, antispasmodic, vulner-ary, antimicrobial, mild sedative.

Pharmacological properties
The anti-inflammatory effect of $(-)$-α-bisabolol, chamazulene, matricine, of a hy-drophilic extract and of the essential oil of Matricaria flower can be demonstrated by various pharmacological models. On an equimolar basis, matricine was found to have a significantly stronger anti-inflammatory ef-fect than chamazulene. The anti-inflamma-tory effect of $(-)$-α-bisabolol is superior to that of chamazulene and of guaiazulene. It is twice as efficient as the synthetic race-mate and $(+)$-α-bisabolol. The results of per-cutaneous administration provide evidence that $(-)$-α-bisabolol is readily absorbed by the skin.
In the croton oil-induced oedema of the mouse ear, apigenin and luteolin were found to have anti-inflammatory activity similar to that of indomethacin. Both flavones gave rise to a pronounced inhibition of leukocyte in-filtration.
Spasms provoked by barium chloride, hist-amine, serotonin, nicotine, bradykinin and oxytocin were inhibited by apigenin. With a titre of 3.29 x papaverine, apigenin was shown to be more effective than papaverine.
The vulnerary action of Matricaria flower or its isolated compounds was demonstrated in studies on the thermally damaged rat tail as well as by the accelerated healing of experi-mentally produced injuries.
Low concentrations of the essential oil have a bacteriostatic and bactericidal effect on gram-positive pathogens and show a remark-able fungicidal action against der-matophytes.
By means of a hexobarbital-induced sleep, spontaneous mobility and explorative activi-ty in mice were tested. A mild sedative effect was shown.

Indications
Internal use:
Gastrointestinal spasms and inflammatory conditions of the gastrointestinal tract; pep-tic ulcers.
Traditionally used for mild sleep disorders, particularly in children.
External use:
Inflammations and irritations of skin and mu-cosa, including the oral cavity and the gums, the respiratory tract and the anal and genital area.

Contra-indications
None known.

Side effects
Extremely rare contact allergy.

Use during pregnancy and lactation
No adverse effects reported.

Special warnings
None required.

Interactions
None reported.

Dosage
Internal:
2 to 3 g of the drug, or as infusion; 1 to 4 ml of tincture (1:5).
Three to four times daily.
Other preparations to be used accordingly.
External:
For compresses, rinses or gargles, 3−10% m/V infusion or approx. 1% V/V alcoholic preparations. For baths 5 g of the drug or 0.8 g of alcoholic preparations per litre of water.
For semi-solid preparations, 3−10% m/m of the drug.

Mode of administration
Oral or topical administration in appropriate dosage forms.

Duration of administration
No restriction.

Overdose
No intoxication symptoms reported.

Effects on ability to drive and use machines
None.

References
See ESCOP Monograph Proposals, Vol. 1 (October 1990)

Menthae piperitae aetheroleum
(Peppermint Oil)

(c) ESCOP – March 1992

Definition
Peppermint oil is obtained by steam distillation from aerial parts of flowering Mentha x piperita L.
It contains not less than 4.5 and not more than 10.0 per cent (m/m) of esters calculated as menthyl acetate ($C_{12}H_{22}O_2$; M_r 198.3), not less than 44.0 per cent (m/m) of free alcohols calculated as menthol ($C_{10}H_{20}O$; M_r 156.3) and not less than 15.0 and not more than 32.0 per cent (m/m) of ketones calculated as menthone ($C_{10}H_{18}O$; M_r 154.3).

The material complies with the European Pharmacopoeia.

Constituents
The main constituent is menthol, mainly in the form of (−)-menthol. The oil also contains menthyl acetate, menthone, menthofuran and small amounts of viridoflorol (which is characteristic for the plant species) and pulegone.

Action
Spasmolytic, carminative, choleretic, antiseptic, refrigerant.

Pharmacological properties
Peppermint oil has a direct spasmolytic action on smooth muscle, especially on that of the intestine. Spasms during endoscopy can be suppressed by application in the colon of a dilute peppermint oil suspension. It also has a choleretic activity, i. e. in enhances the production of bile.

Two actions in the respiratory tract are reported: secretolytic in the bronchi and decongestant in the nose. However, the relief of complaints caused by common cold by inhalation or application in the mouth of peppermint oil is probably caused by stimulation of the cold receptors in the respiratory tract, which gives a feeling of easier respiration.

Application of peppermint oil in low doses causes a decrease in the sensitivity of the nerve receptors and some inhibition of nerve conduction; higher doses cause a transient stimulation of the sensory nerves and receptors. Cold receptors, however, are stimulated by low doses.

Menthol inhibits the de novo synthesis of cholesterol and fatty acids in the liver, resulting in the dissolution of cholesterol gall stones.

Some antiseptic activity has been reported; in otolaryngeal infections it is not efficacious, although not objectionable.

Indications
Internal use: spastic conditions of the upper gastrointestinal tract and bile ducts; gall bladder inflammation; gall stones; flatulence; symptomatic treatment of irritable bowel syndrome; catarrh of the respiratory tract.

External use: inflammation of the oral mucosa; rheumatic conditions; local muscle and nerve pain; skin conditions such as pruritus and urticaria.
Traditionally used as an expectorant.

Contra-indications
Hypersensitivity to peppermint oil.

Side effects
Extremely rare. Few cases of skin irritation are reported; in single cases the use of oil, not contained in enteric-coated capsules, caused heartburn, especially in person suffering from reflux oesophagitis.

Use during pregnancy and lactation
No adverse effects reported.

Special warnings
In case of bile duct obstruction, gall stones or gall bladder inflammation a physician must be consulted.
In the treatment of irritable bowel syndrome peppermint oil must be administered in enteric-coated capsules to avoid stomach irritation and heartburn.
Application of peppermint oil (preparations) in as well as on or around the nose of babies and small children must be avoided (because of the risk, among others, of laryngeal and bronchial spasms). Inhalation of menthol may also cause bronchial obstruction in older children and adults.
Menthol can cause jaundice in neonates compromised by glucose-6-phosphate dehydrogenase deficiency.

Interactions
Patients with achlorhydria (as caused by medication with H_2 receptor blockers such as cimetidine and ranitidine) should use peppermint oil only in enteric-coated capsules.

Dosage
Unless otherwise prescribed:
Internal use:
Average daily dose: 0.2−0.4 ml.
− For inhalation: 3−4 drops added to hot water or as a lozenge containing 2−10 mg.
− For irritable bowel syndrome: average single dose 0.2−0.4 ml; average daily dose 0.6−1.2 ml, preferably enteric-coated.

External sue:
− Diluted oil (0.2−1%) rubbed into the affected area.
− Preparations (content 0.2−1%) are used similarly.

Mode of administration
Internally: as diluted oil, in enteric-coated capsules or in suppositories, or as inhalations.
Externally: as diluted oil or in galenical preparations.

Duration of administration
No adverse effects from long term use are known (see however: Overdose).

Overdose
Overdoses (more than 4 g day) produce a general sensation of cold, stomach ache, cardiac problems, ataxia and other CNS problems caused by the presence of menthol.

Effects on ability to drive and use machines
Nothing reported.

References
See ESCOP Monograph Proposals, Vol. 3 (March 1992)

Passiflorae herba
(Passiflora)

(c) ESCOP – March 1992

Definition
Passiflora consists of the dried aerial parts bearing flowers or fruits of *Passiflora incarnata* L. It contains not less than 0.3 per cent of flavonoids, calculated as hyperoside ($C_{21}H_{20}O_{12}$, M_r 464.4), or not less than 0.8 per cent of total flavonoids, calculated as vitexin ($C_{21}H_{20}O_{10}$, M_r 432.4).
The material complies with the French or German or Swiss pharmacopoeias.
Fresh material may also be used provided that when dried it complies with one of the above pharmacopoeias.

Constituents
Flavonoids, mainly C-glycosides of apigenin and luteolin, e. g. schaftoside, isoschaftoside

and the 2"-β-D-glucosides of isovitexin and isoorientin; a small amount of maltol; traces of essential oil and a cyanogenic glycoside; possibly traces of indole alkaloids depending on the origin and maturity of the plant.

Action
Sedative, anxiolytic

Pharmacological properties
Passiflora showed a sedative effect in rodents.

On i.p. injection Passiflora extract reduced the spontaneous locomotor activity in mice and prolonged the sleeping time.

The nociceptive threshold was raised in different test models and also after oral administration.

Rats showed reduced general activity on prolonged treatment with Passiflora extract.

Passiflora extracts show papaverine-like spasmolytic effects.

In one study an anxiolytic effect of Passiflora was observed whereas the locomotor activity remained unaffected.

Maltol isolated from Passiflora inhibited spontaneous motor activity in mice and prolonged the hexobarbital sleeping time. The effective doses were however far beyond the amounts normally administered with Passiflora preparations.

It is not clear which constituents are responsible for the actions of Passiflora.

Indications
Nervous tension, particularly in cases of sleep disturbance or exaggerated awareness of heartbeat (palpitations)

Contra-indications
None known.

Side effects
None known.

Use during pregnancy and lactation
No adverse effects reported.

Special warnings
None required.

Interactions
None reported.

Dosage
0.5 to 2 g of the drug; 2.5 g of drug as infusion; 1 to 4 ml of tincture [1 : 10] three to four times daily. Other preparations accordingly.

Mode of administration
Oral, in liquid or solid dosage forms.

Duration of administration
No restriction.

Overdose
Nothing reported; neither dependence nor withdrawal symptoms are reported.

Effects on ability to drive and use machines
Nothing reported.

References
See ESCOP Monograph Proposals, Vol. 2 (March 1992)

Plantaginis ovatae semen
(Ispaghula)

(c) ESCOP – March 1992

Definition
Ispaghula consists of the ripe seeds of *Plantago ovata* Forsskal [*Plantago ispaghula* Roxburgh] including the husk, with a swelling index of not less than 9.

The material complies with Deutsches Arzneibuch.

Constituents
As main active constituents the seeds contain about 80 per cent of total dietary fibre when determined by the AOAC method, consisting predominantly of insoluble fibre. Soluble fibre occurs in the epidermis, as mucilage polysaccharide consisting mainly of a highly branched arabinoxylan with a xylan backbone and branches of arabinose, xylose and galacturonic acid-rhamnose. The seeds also contain proteins, starch, fixed oil, sterols and the trisaccharide planteose.

Action
Bowel function regulator.

Pharmacological properties

(i) Bulk forming laxative.

Increases the volume of intestinal contents by binding of fluid which leads to a physical stimulation of the gut wall. The intraluminal pressure is decreased and colon transit is accelerated.

Increases stool weight and stool water content by fibre residue, by water bound to the residue and by increased faecal bacterial mass.

(ii) Antidiarrhoeal effects.

Increases the viscosity of intestinal contents by binding of fluid.

Prolongs transit time by increased viscosity of contents, thus normalizing defecation frequency.

(iii) Metabolic effects.

Lowers blood cholesterol levels by binding bile acids and increasing their faecal excretion which, in turn, results in further bile salt synthesis from cholesterol.

Reduces peak levels of blood glucose by delaying intestinal absorption of sugar.

(iv) Mucosa-protective effects.

Decreases the β-glucuronidase activity of colon bacteria, thus inhibiting the cleavage of toxic compounds from their liver conjugates.

Reduced bacterial conversion of primary bile acids to the more toxic secondary ones has been observed.

Short-chain fatty acids (acetate, propionate, butyrate) released from the digestible part of the fibre by bacterial fermentation have a trophic and differentiating effect on the mucosal cells.

Indications

Habitual constipation; conditions in which easy defecation with soft motions is desirable, e.g. anal fissures, haemorrhoids, after rectal surgery and in pregnancy. For conditioning of the intestine in irregular motions: Irritable bowel syndrome, diverticulosis. To maintain normal bowel functions in fibre deficient diets, e.g. in weight reduction. Adjuvant therapy for diarrhoea of various origins.

Contra-indications

Stenoses of the gastro-intestinal tract; ileus. Diabetes mellitus where insulin adjustment is difficult.

Side effects

In rare cases hypersensitivity reactions may occur.

Use during pregnancy and lactation

No adverse effects reported.

Special warnings

None required.

Interactions

The absorption of drugs taken at the same time can be delayed. Insulin dependent diabetics may need less insulin due to retarded absorption of glucose.

Dosage

Adult daily dose as a laxative: 7 to 30 g of the seeds or equivalent preparations; in cases of diarrhoea, up to 40 g.

Children: according to age and body weight.

Mode of administration

For oral administration only, as whole seeds, or other preparations.

It is important to take the seeds with a large amount of liquid, e.g. 200 ml of water to 5 g of the drug.

The seeds should be taken 0.5−1 hour after intake of other drugs.

Duration of administration

No adverse effects from long term use are known.

A doctor should be consulted if diarrhoea lasts more than 3 days.

Overdose

No toxic effects reported.

Effects on ability to drive and use machines

Nothing reported.

References

See ESCOP Monograph Proposals, Vol. 2 (March 1992)

Sennae folium
(Senna Leaf)

(c) ESCOP – October 1990

Definition
Senna leaf consists of the dried leaflets of *Cassia senna* L. [*C. acutifolia* Delile], known as Alexandrian or Khartoum senna, or *Cassia angustifolia* Vahl, known as Tinnevelly senna, or a mixture of the leaflets of the two species. It contains not less than 2.5 per cent of hydroxyanthracene glycosides, calculated as sennoside B (M_r 863).
The material complies with the European Pharmacopoeia.

Constituents
The main active constituents are sennosides A and B which are rhein-dianthrone diglucosides. There are also small quantities of other dianthrone diglucosides, monoanthraquinone glucosides and aglycones.

Action
Laxative.

Pharmacological properties
1.8-dihydroxyanthracene derivatives possess a laxative effect. The β-linked glucosides (sennosides) are prodrugs which are not absorbed in the upper gut and which act specifically on the colon after having been converted into the active metabolite (rheinanthrone) by the microflora of the large intestine.
There are two different mechanisms of action:
- an influence on the motility of the large intestine (stimulation of peristaltic contractions and inhibition of local contractions) resulting in an accelerated colonic transit, thus reducing fluid absorption.
- an influence on secretion processes (stimulation of mucus and active chloride secretion) resulting in enhanced fluid secretion.
The motility effects are mediated by direct stimulation of colonic neurons and possibly by prostaglandins. In the secretory effect, Ca^{2+}, prostaglandins and neurohumoral mechanisms are involved as mediators.

Defecation takes place after a delay of several hours (8–12 hours) due to the time taken for transport to the colon and metabolization into the active compound.

Indications
Constipation and all cases in which easy defecation with soft faeces is desirable, e.g. in cases of anal fissures, haemorrhoids and after rectal and abdominal surgery, as well as for bowel clearance before surgery and in diagnostic investigations.

Contra-indications
Inflammatory colon disases (e.g. ulcerative colitis, Crohn's disease), ileus, appendicitis, abdominal pain of unknown origin.

Side effects
If used correctly, side effects will be minimal.
- Sensitive individuals may occasionally experience abdominal spasms or diarrhoea and should reduce their dose.
- Yellow or red (pH-dependent) discoloration of urine by metabolites, which is harmless.
- Chronic use may cause pigmentation of the colon (pseudomelanosis coli), which is harmless and reversible after drug discontinuation.

Use during pregnancy and lactation
Senna may be used during pregnancy and lactation in the prescribed dosage range. There is no evidence for stimulation of uterine activity or any embryotoxic effect. Although traces of metabolites appear in breast milk, the amounts are far too low to induce a laxative effect in the nursed infant.

Special warnings
Long term use of laxatives should be avoided. Abuse, with consequent fluid and electrolyte losses, may cause:
- dependence with possible need for increased dosages,
- disturbance of the water and electrolyte balance (mainly hypokalemia),
- an atonic colon with impaired function.

Interactions
Hypokalaemia (resulting from long term laxative abuse) potentiates the action of cardiac

glycosides and interacts with antiarrhythmic drugs, with drugs which induce reversion to sinus rhythm (e. g. quinidine) and with other drugs which induce hypokalemia (e. g. corticoids, diuretics).

Dosage

Adult daily dose: drug equivalent to 10−60 mg of hydroxyanthracene derivatives calculated as sennoside B; for bowel clearance 120−160 mg in a single dose.
Children from 6 to 12 years: half of the adult dosage.

Mode of administration

For oral administration only, in liquid or solid dosage forms.

Duration of administration

Should not be taken for long periods.

Overdose

The major symptoms are griping and severe diarrhoea with consequent losses of fluid and electrolyte, which should be replaced.

Effects on ability to drive and use machines

None.

References

See ESCOP Monograph Proposals, Vol. 1 (October 1990)

Sennae fructus acutifoliae
(Alexandrian Senna Pods)

Sennae fructus angustifoliae
(Tinnevelly Senna Pods)

(c) ESCOP – October 1990

Definition

Alexandrian senna pods consists of the dried fruit of *Cassia senna* L. [*C. acutifolia* Delile]. It contains not less than 3.4 per cent of hydroxyanthracene glycosides, calculated as sennoside B (M_r 863).
Tinnevelly senna pods consists of the dried fruit of *Cassia angustifolia* Vahl. It contains not less than 2.2 per cent of hydroxyanthracene glycosides, calculated as sennoside B (M_r 863).

Both materials comply with the European Pharmacopoeia.

Constituents

The main active constituents are sennosides A and B which are rhein-dianthrone diglucosides. There are also small quantities of other dianthrone diglucosides, monoanthraquinone glucosides and aglycones.

Action

Laxative.

Pharmacological properties

1,8-dihydroxyanthracene derivatives possess a laxative effect. The β-linked glucosides (sennosides) are prodrugs which are not absorbed in the upper gut and which act specifically on the colon after having been converted into the active metabolite (rheinanthrone) by the microflora of the large intestine.
There are two different mechanisms of action:
− an influence on the motility of the large intestine (stimulation of peristaltic contractions and inhibition of local contractions) resulting in an accelerated colonic transit, thus reducing fluid absorption.
− an influence on secretion processes (stimulation of mucus and active chloride secretion) resulting in enhanced fluid secretion.
The motility effects are mediated by direct stimulation of colonic neurons and possibly by prostaglandins. In the secretory effect, Ca^{2+}, prostaglandins and neurohumoral mechanisms are involved as mediators.
Defecation takes place after a delay of several hours (8−12 hours) due to the time taken for transport to the colon and metabolization into the active compund.

Indications

Constipation and all cases in which easy defecation with soft faeces is desirable, e. g. in cases of anal fissures, haemorrhoids and after rectal and abdominal surgery, as well as for bowel clearance before surgery and in diagnostic investigations.

Contra-indications

Inflammatory colon diseases (e. g. ulcerative colitis, Crohn's disease), ileus, appendicitis, abdominal pain of unknown origin.

Side effects

If used correctly, side effects will be minimal. Sensitive individuals may occasionally experience abdominal spasms or diarrhoea and should reduce their dose.

- Yellow or red (pH-dependent) discoloration of urine by metabolites, which is harmless.
- Chronic use may cause pigmentation of the colon (pseudomelanosis coli), which is harmless and reversible after drug discontinuation.

Special warnings

Long term use of laxatives should be avoided. Abuse, with consequent fluid and electrolyte losses, may cause:
- dependence with possible need for increased dosages,
- disturbance of the water and electrolyte balance (mainly hypokalemia),
- an atonic colon with impaired function.

Use during pregnancy and lactation

Senna may be used during pregnancy and lactation in the prescribed dosage range. There is no evidence for stimulation of uterine activity or any embryotoxic effect.

Although traces of metabolites appear in breast milk, the amounts are far too low to induce a laxative effect in the nursed infant.

Interactions

Hypokalemia (resulting from long term laxative abuse) potentiates the action of cardiac glycosides and interacts with antiarrhythmic drugs, with drugs which induce reversion to sinus rhythm (e.g. quinidine) and with other drugs which induce hypokalemia (e.g. corticoids, diuretics).

Dosage

Adult daily dose: drug equivalent to 10−60 mg of hydroxyanthracene derivatives calculated as sennoside B; for bowel clearance 120−160 mg in a single dose.

Children from 6 to 12 years: half of the adult dosage.

Mode of administration

For oral administration only, in liquid or solid dosage forms.

Duration of administration

Should not be taken for long periods.

Overdose

The major symptoms are griping and severe diarrhoea with consequent losses of fluid and electrolyte, which should be replaced.

Effects on ability to drive and use machines

None.

References

See ESCOP Monograph Proposals, Vol. 1 (October 1990)

Taraxaci folium
(Dandelion Leaf)

(c) ESCOP – March 1992

Definition

Dandelion leaf consists of the dried leaves of *Taraxacum officinale* Wiggers, *s.s.* (*T. officinale* Weber, *s.l.*), collected before flowering.

The material complies with the British Herbal Pharmacopoeia.

Fresh material may also be used provided that when dried it complies with the British Herbal Pharmacopoeia.

Constituents

Sesquiterpene lactones of the germacranolide type, as glucosides; triterpenes such as cycloartenol; phytosterols; p-hydroxyphenylacetic acid; minerals, especially potassium (about 4% in dried leaf).

Action

Diuretic, choleretic.

Pharmacological properties

In experiments on mice and rats the diuretic and saluretic indices of a fluid extract of Dandelion herb, corresponding to approximately 8 g dried herb/kg body weight, are greater than those of Dandelion root and comparable to those of furosemide (80 mg/kg body weight). The high potassium content of the herb ensures replacement of potassium eliminated in the urine.

The principal bitter constituents of the leaf are the sesquiterpene lactones taraxinic acid glucoside and its 11,13-dihydro derivative, which may produce the choleretic action. These and other bitter tasting compounds are also present in dandelion root, which increases bile secretion in rats by over 40%.

Indications
Water retention due to various causes.

Contra-indications
Occlusion of the bile ducts; gall-bladder empyema; ileus.

Side effects
No adverse effects confirmed.

Use during pregnancy and lactation
No adverse effects reported.

Special warnings
None required.

Interactions
None reported.

Dosage
4–10 g of the drug, or as an infusion, 3 times daily;
2–5 ml of tincture (1:5) in 25% ethanol, 3 times daily;
5–10 ml of juice from fresh leaf, twice daily; other equivalent preparations.

Mode of administration
Oral.

Duration of administration
No adverse effects from long term use are known.

Overdose
No toxic effects reported.

Effects on ability to drive and use machines
Nothing reported

References
See ESCOP Monograph Proposals, Vol. 3 (March 1992)

Taraxaci radix
(Dandelion Root)

(c) ESCOP – March 1992

Definition
Dandelion root consists of the dried root and rhizome of *Taraxacum officinale* Wiggers, *s. s.* (*T. officinale* Weber, *s. l.*).
The material complies with the Österreichisches Arzneibuch and the British Herbal Pharmacopoeia.
Fresh material may also be used provided that when dried it complies with one of the above mentioned pharmacopoeias.

Constituents
Sesquiterpene lactones of the eudesmanolide and germacranolide types; triterpene alcohols and phytosterols; phenolic compounds: taraxacoside, caffeic acid and p-hydroxyphenylacetic acid; potassium. In autumn the dried root contains up to 40% inulin, in spring about 2%.

Action
Digestive stimulant, cholagogue, choleretic.

Pharmacological properties
An alcoholic extract of the whole plant is choleretic – the bile secretion in rats increases by over 40%.
The bitter tasting compounds are thought to cause stimulation of the digestion.
A mild laxative action is reported.
The traditional use for rheumatic conditions could be related to the moderate anti-inflammatory activity of Dandelion root observed in rats.

Indications
Hepatobiliary disorders, dyspepsia, loss of appetite.
Traditionally for relief of rheumatic disorders.

Contra-indications
Occlusion of the bile ducts, gall-bladder empyema; ileus.

Side effects
No adverse effects confirmed.

Use during pregnancy and lactation
No adverse effects reported.

Special warnings
None required.

Interactions
None reported.

Dosage
3 g of the drug or 5−10 ml of the tincture (1 : 5) in 25% ethanol; other equivalent preparations.

Mode of administration
Oral.

Duration of administration
No adverse effects from long term use are known.

Overdose
No toxic effects reported.

Effects on ability to drive and use machines
Nothing reported.

References
See ESCOP Monograph Proposals, Vol. 3 (March 1992)

Uvae ursi folium
Uva Ursi (Bearberry Leaf)

(c) ESCOP – March 1992

Definition
Uva Ursi consists of the dried leaves of *Arctostaphylos uva-ursi* (L.) Sprengel. It contains not less than 6.0 per cent of hydroquinone derivatives calculated as anhydrous arbutin ($C_{12}H_{16}O_7$, M_r 272.3).
The material complies with the French, German or Swiss pharmacopoeias.

Constituents
Hydroquinone derivatives, principally arbutin and a smaller amount of methylarbutin; polyphenols (tannins) including galloyl esters of arbutin; piceoside, a phenolic glucoside; flavonoids, mainly glycosides of quercetin and myricetin; monotropein, an iridoid glycoside; triterpenes including ursolic acid, uvaol and amyrin derivatives.

Action
Urinary antiseptic; astringent.

Pharmacological properties
In the lower intestine arbutin is enzymatically hydrolysed and the aglycone, hydroquinone, probably provides the ultimate antibacterial action of uva ursi (at an optimum pH below 7). The hydroquinone is metabolized to glucuronide and sulphate esters.
Based on in vitro results it is debatable whether the antibacterial activity is due to the hydroquinone sulphate ester or to the free hydroquinone. Cleavage of the ester is possible by saponification in urine of alkaline pH (ca. pH 8) or may be due to the action of enzymes from the microorganisms causing the infection.
The high tannin content of uva ursi causes the astringent effect.

Indications
Mild infections of the urinary tract.

Contra-indications
Sensitive stomach conditions; kidney disorders.

Side effects
Nausea and vomiting may occur.

Use during pregnancy and lactation
No adverse effects reported.
As with all medicines for which no specific data is available caution should be exercised particularly during the first three months of pregnancy.

Special warnings
None required.

Interactions
None reported.

Dosage
1.5−2.5 of the drug, or as infusion or as cold aqueous extract.
Other equivalent preparations 3 to 4 times daily.

Mode of administration
Oral.

Duration of administration
Treatment should be of short duration (not more than 7 days).
Extensive use over long periods could lead to disturbance of the liver function.

Overdose
The major symptoms would be acute stomach upset and liver damage.

Effects on ability to drive and use machines
Nothing reported.

References
See ESCOP Monograph Proposals, Vol. 3 (March 1992).

Valerianae radix
(Valerian Root)

(c) ESCOP – October 1990

Definition
Valerian root consists of the subterranean organs of *Valeriana officinalis* L. s. l. including the rhizome, roots and stolons, carefully dried at a temperature below 40 °C. It contains not less than 0,5 per cent V/m of essential oil.
The material complies with the European Pharmacopoeia.
Fresh material may also be used provided that when dried it complies with the European Pharmacopoeia.

Constituents
Essential oil with monoterpenes and sesquiterpenes, mainly valerenic acids; up to 1 per cent thermo- and chemolabile valepotriates.

Action
Sedative, spasmolytic, relaxant.

Pharmacological properties
Various constituents appear to contribute to the sedative and relaxant effects of the drug. An aqueous extract as well as a tincture reduced spontaneous motility in mice.
In a pharmacological screening test the sesquiterpenoids valeranone and valerenic acid, both components of the essential oil, exerted a central depressant and muscle relaxant effect. Valerenic acid influenced the locomotility of mice in a similar way to pentobarbital.
It has been suggested that certain constituents of Valeriana officinalis interact with the metabolism of gamma-aminobutyric acid in the brain. Another study indicates the interaction of hydroalcoholic extract with receptors mediating sedation in the central nervous system. Even the strong odour may contribute to the calming effect.
Valeriana officinalis preparations are considered as safe despite the known in vitro alkylating activity of the valepotriates which has been attributed to their epoxide structure. This is because valepotriates decompose rapidly in the stored drug and, if detectable in preparations, only traces of valepotriates or their degradation products (in part, baldrinals) are normally found.
Furthermore, valepotriates are badly absorbed from the gastro-intestinal tract.

Indications
Nervous tension, excitability, restlessness and sleep disturbances.
Traditionally used also for stress and anxiety states.

Contra-indications
None known.

Side effects
No adverse effects confirmed.

Use during pregnancy and lactation
No adverse effects reported.

Special warnings
None required.

Interactions
None reported.

Dosage
Adults: 1 to 3 g of the drug (e. g. as a tea) up to three times daily or 1 to 3 ml of tincture (1:5) up to three times daily; other preparations equivalent.
Children: according to age and bodyweight.

Mode of administration
Oral, in liquid or solid dosage forms.
Externally, as a bath additive.

Duration of administration

No restriction, neither dependence nor withdrawal symptoms are reported.

Overdose

No intoxication symptoms reported.

Effects on ability to drive and use machines

Nothing reported.

References

See ESCOP Monograph Proposals, Vol. 1 (October 1990).

Subject Index